HARVARD BOOKS
IN BIOLOGY

Number 3

THE INTEGRITY
OF THE BODY

The Integrity
of the Body

A Discussion of Modern Immunological Ideas

F. M. BURNET, F.R.S.

The Walter and Eliza Hall Institute
of Medical Research, Melbourne, Australia

HARVARD UNIVERSITY PRESS

Cambridge · 1962

Distributed in Great Britain by Oxford University Press, London

Library of Congress Catalog Card Number 62–8180
Printed in the United States of America

Preface

It is always difficult to say for whom a book is written or why it is written at all. If I had to answer such an inquiry about this one, I should probably say that it was written primarily to provide the information about immunology that I should like to have if I were a botanist or a geneticist or a physician with the same avid curiosity about things as they are that I have as a microbiologist. And there is an important secondary reason. I am not a university teacher but I know that there is no better way to clarify one's understanding of one's own subject than to expound it in the simplest possible terms. All academics, whether they are teachers or not, must be enthusiastic about their hobby and must have an audience on which they can test their flash of insight, however tiny it is.

In these pages I have taken the point of view that immunity has aspects deeper and more interesting than those concerned simply with defense against infectious disease. In its broadest sense it seems to be part of the processes by which the structural and functional integrity of every complex organism is maintained. This theme of immunity as based on the demand for chemical and cellular consistency within the body is the essence of the book. I have been concerned with immunology for more than 35 years and during that period I have been specially interested in watching the subject emerge from its little medical niche into a significant relation to biology as a whole.

At the present time there is a specially active interest in immunology among those whose work impinges on the theoretical foundations of biology. Geneticists and biochemists have realized the special potentialities of antibodies as biologically labeled proteins to throw light on the process by which genetic information carried in the chromosomes is eventually manifested in the synthesis of the functional proteins needed for the functioning of the organism. In addition, there are many specialized applications of immunology in the other biological sciences.

It is hoped that this outline of the facts and theories of immunity may be useful to biologists generally — including those applied biologists, physicians, surgeons, veterinarians, and animal breeders — as well as those for whom an interest in biology is without professional bias. An elementary knowledge of chemistry and biology has been assumed in the reader but no special familiarity with medicine or the medical sciences.

F. M. B.

Contents

The Integrity
of the Body

1. Historical Outline

The story of immunity goes back to antiquity. It is probable that for as long as such characteristic diseases of children as chickenpox, measles, and mumps have existed mothers and nurses must have known that one attack only was the rule. Smallpox was a matter of more importance and it seems likely that it was the unique character of smallpox in leaving unmistakable evidence of its attack — the pock-marked face — which provided the beginning of systematic thought on immunity. No man with a pock-marked face suffered again from smallpox, no matter how severe the epidemic. Implicit in this observation are the two basic doctrines of infectious disease, that each is due to a specific microorganism and that postinfectious immunity is also specific. It is no accident that experimental work on immunology, and for that matter on virology, dates from Jenner's famous experiment with "matter" from the finger of the dairymaid, Sarah Phelps.

There were other ways in which the workings of immunity could be recognized in the era before biological experimentation was possible. In the 17th, 18th, and 19th centuries it was well known to every administrator, admiral, or general with responsibilities in the West Indies or on the West coast of Africa that men newly arrived from Europe suffered a terrifying mortality from yellow fever, but that natives of the country, including Europeans brought up there from childhood, were unaffected.

The impossibility of differentiating clearly between yellow fever, malaria, and the other tropical fevers left the nature of this immunity uncertain. Most writers of the time referred to the resistance to disease provided by acclimatization, and some believed that the important aspect of acclimatization was to have been fortunate enough to have survived an attack of yellow fever. It was known that yellow fever was on the average much milder in children than in adults of the same race. In the very first epidemic of yellow fever on the North American continent, at Yucatan in 1648, it was recorded that: "The robust, young, and healthy died first. Of those of tender age attacked, few died as compared with adults and the aged. God spared the young and innocent but not the sinful elders."

Those who are old enough to remember the great influenza epidemic of 1918–19 will know that then, too, the main incidence of death was on the robust and healthy — the young male adult as against children and those over 40.

All through this book the emphasis will be on the integration of immunology into the pattern of general biology as viewed from the evolutionary standpoint. The first point we need to be sure about is that immunity is something that has had a significant effect on survival in the past — that it has been molded under specific evolutionary pressures and is not something that has emerged more or less accidentally in connection with some only distantly related bodily function or evolutionary requirement. If it is a general rule that the *first* impact of an infectious disease is more likely to kill if it takes place in adult life than if it is experienced in early childhood, we have an immediate and powerful indication of the importance of immunity for survival. In the case of a disease like yellow fever, we have the additional advantage that may be conveyed by maternal immunity. A child is born carrying immunity obtained from its mother's blood. In general this immunity fades to an insignificant level within a year, but in an environment where infection is nearly universal many children would suffer first infection while they were still partly immune and perhaps reach their full personal immunity without any visible illness whatever.

When we say that the processes of immunity have evolved as something helpful to survival, we encounter an interesting difficulty, namely, that men, like most gregarious animals, are subject to a wide range of parasitic disease. There is very little in common among the organisms which produce yellow fever, syphilis, tuberculosis, ringworm, and trichinosis, nor is it conceivable that the best way of countering the effect of one type of infection is the best way for dealing with all the others. In the course of evolution, then, nature has obviously had to accept compromises in order to produce the type of immune mechanism which provided the best over-all chance of survival under the average circumstances. Most of our interest is directed toward our own species and I have often wondered whether the main factor which shaped our immunological evolution might not have been the tropical arboreal life of our distant ancestors. If we can judge from the distribution and habits of their present prototypes, the major part of human evolution took place in tropical jungles. Orthodox opinion traces development from some early small mammal of unspecialized type through forms roughly equivalent to tree shrew, lemur, monkey, and anthropoid ape to man. At all stages there would have been exposure to infection by the viruses and protozoa transmitted by mosquitoes and similar biting insects. Since none of the prototypes of our ancestors are truly gregarious but move about in family groups or small bands, there would have been little scope for infectious disease to spread by personal contact. Measles under modern conditions can persist only in large communities and could neither have developed nor survived among small isolated groups. It is possible, therefore, that it is no accident that yellow fever comes first to mind when we seek an evolutionary justification for what we find in the study of immunity. Yellow fever, like other diseases carried by free-flying insects and not restricted to only one species of host, would be the type of infection most likely to involve rather rare animals dwelling in tropical forests. It is the perfect example of the sorts of infection that must have persisted over the whole evolutionary history of man as a mammal.

There is another aspect of evolution which must always be kept in mind: that adaptations must make use of available potentialities. Whatever the demands for protection against microorganisms, they had to be fulfilled within the limitations of an organism with a predetermined pattern of biochemical function, with blood vessels and circulation of vertebrate type, and with strictly limited powers of regenerating cells and tissues lost or irretrievably damaged by disease or violence. Ideally we could hope to provide a self-consistent picture of how the immune processes fit into the day-to-day functioning of the human body and how this integration has developed in the course of evolution. We are still far from achieving this objective. As in most fields of biology, there is no grand design against which we can arrange the various aspects of immunity that thrust themselves on our attention in real life or emerge in the laboratory. Some form of general concept will always be needed, however, and there *are* general theories of immunity, some of which we shall discuss. It will be very easy to see, however, that none of the theories are adequate. In all there is an *ad hoc* element relevant to nothing but our present conception of the facts of immunity.

To return to the historical significance of smallpox and the first attempts to immunize against it, in 18th-century England smallpox was the most important of the diseases of childhood, and among the upper classes there was much interest in the method of variolation, brought from Constantinople by a famous bluestocking, Lady Mary Wortley Montagu. This involved inoculation of children on the skin with "matter" from a pustule of a mild case of smallpox. In most instances the child in its turn showed mild symptoms, with only a few scattered pocks, and was subsequently immune. Variolation was being widely discussed in cultivated circles at the end of the 18th century and the time was ripe for Jenner to pay attention to folk tales from Gloucestershire that dairymaids were immune to smallpox. He checked the observation in a very brief series of experiments, probably the first set investigation in experimental immunology. Jenner's experiment is immortal, but it is well to remember that it was a scrappy experiment. When Jenner submitted an account for publication in the *Philosophical Transactions* of the Royal Society, the editors, probably rightly, considered that the evidence for his sweeping claims was insufficient and refused to publish it. Jenner published his own report, became famous, and spent the rest of his life in controversies over priority and rewards. The history of vaccination is not particularly edifying, and to this day it is uncertain whether the virus we now use for vaccination against smallpox is descended from Jenner's cowpox virus or from smallpox virus which had accidentally been transferred from child to child at some period. Nevertheless it is a fact that *pari passu* with the extension of vaccination, smallpox rapidly became relatively unimportant in Europe, measles taking its place as the main cause of death from infectious disease in childhood. By 1859 the principle that a mild form of a given infection could protect against the virulent natural form had been firmly implanted in medical thought.

With the emergence of the new science of medical bacteriology from the researches of Pasteur, Koch, and their contemporaries, it was inevitable that the same principle should be applied to other infections. Pasteur made the first step in studying chicken cholera, a bacterial disease of fowls due to *Pasteurella avisepticus*. The bacterium grows readily in a simple chicken broth and the injection of very small doses of pure culture is fatal to unprotected chickens. Pasteur found that chickens inoculated from very old cultures that had been left for some months untouched showed mild or no symptoms and recovered. Whether by accident or by inspiration, such recovered fowls were later inoculated with virulent culture and survived. Pasteur soon established the regularity of such a result and spent the rest of his scientific career in working out similar methods for the "attenuation" of the pathogenic bacteria or viruses responsible for anthrax, swine erysipelas, and rabies. This approach has continued right up to the present. Perhaps the most important modifications of the Pasteurian approach have been the use of killed bacteria or virus to produce an imitation of a mild infection and the development of a genetic approach to produce satisfactorily attenuated cultures of the infectious agent. Neither of these topics is directly relevant to an understanding of the nature of immunity and it is more rewarding to follow the more academic experiments which aimed at elucidating the actual process by which protection was afforded.

During the 1880's, two opposing concepts emerged. One

group of workers found that blood serum had power to kill certain bacteria. At first, attention was concentrated on the bactericidal power of normal serum, but it gradually became clear that after experimental infection with a bacterial culture the animal's serum often developed new properties. Sometimes there was an actively destructive effect on the culture, sometimes the bacteria were agglutinated without being killed. These new properties began to be ascribed to a group of substances at first wholly hypothetical, the antibodies. Experiments soon showed that the antibodies which developed after experimental infection with bacteria were specific; they clumped or destroyed only bacteria of the type that had produced the infection. It was natural that workers interested in antibodies grew to feel that they were of special importance in immunity to disease. Another group, led by Metchnikoff, was more impressed with the power of certain white cells of blood and other body fluids to take in and destroy bacteria. Eventually, as is so often the case, both groups turned out to be right, and by about 1920 it was accepted that defense against bacterial infection was in the last analysis the function of the white blood cells, the phagocytes which eat and destroy bacteria, but that their activities were greatly helped if antibody from the serum of an immune animal was attached to the bacterial surface.

Nowadays, with the universal use of sulfonamides and antibiotics, interest in the finer details of immunity against bacteria has become sporadic. There is still much to be found out, but it is work of little human significance and few are now undertaking it. We are not likely to see another phase of research on bacterial immunity that could rival the wonderful years of research on pneumococcal infection and immunity that Avery guided at the Rockefeller Institute between 1917 and 1942.

Since the advent of sulfapyridine and penicillin, lobar pneumonia has almost vanished from medicine, but it is not so long ago that Osler called it the Captain of the men of Death. Forty years ago every medical ward in a teaching hospital would have a few patients with severe pneumonia, with half the substance of their lung out of action and with high fever. Twenty percent of these patients died. The need to understand the nature of pneumonia and to find means of overcoming it was perhaps the biggest stimulus to research in infectious disease during the 1920's. The organism responsible, the pneumococcus, was well known. The problem was to find out how it first overcame the natural defenses of the lung and then, if the patient was fortunate, how it was subsequently defeated by the new defenses that were brought to bear as immunity developed. To condense a quarter of a century of discovery into a few sentences, we may say that the central feature was the recognition of the importance of the capsular substance of the pneumococcus. This is a semisoluble polysaccharide of gumlike character whose pattern determines the immunological "type" of the organism and which dominates the process of infection and recovery. Antibody, if it is to be effective, must correspond to the type of infecting pneumococcus. In the course of infection much of the capsular material is released from the multiplying pneumococci and the first function of antibody is to mop up all this free antigen. Only then can it coat the surface of the pneumococci themselves, so making it possible for active phagocytosis by white cells to take place. In the old days the onset of effective immune action marked the "crisis," the traditional turning point of acute pneumonia.

Immunity has always been thought of primarily for its medical implications, and another impetus to its development came with the recognition that some bacteria produced symptoms and death because they liberated soluble and diffusible toxins in the body. The classical examples are diphtheria, tetanus, and botulism. In 1890 it was shown by Behring and Kitasato that antitoxins could be produced that neutralized the soluble toxins. This was the first step toward a more sophisticated chemically biased approach to immunity. Ehrlich soon became the dominant figure in the field and his quantitative studies on diphtheria toxin and antitoxin provided the first substantial material on which general ideas about immunity could be based. Ehrlich's own side-chain theory of immunity was the first well-reasoned attempt to do this. He was primarily an organic chemist and was impressed particularly with the quantitative regularity that allowed reasonably accurate titration of toxin and antitoxin. Everything pointed to the conclusions (1) that entry of toxin into the body stimulated it to produce the counteragent antitoxin and (2) that antitoxin combined chemically with toxin, so neutralizing its activity. Ehrlich added a third postulate, that toxin produced its lethal effect by combining with cell substance by means of "side chains" of the giant molecules that were at that time supposed to make up protoplasm. If too many of these side chains were blocked, the cell's nutrition became impossible and death occurred. If exposure to toxin was gradual, Ehrlich believed that there would be an overproduction of these side chains to compensate for the physiological deficiency and that many of these excess side chains were set free in the blood, where they appeared as antitoxin. None of the background assumptions of the side-chain theory are valid today and nothing would be gained by elaborating and refuting Ehrlich's arguments. Nevertheless there is one aspect of the theory that it is important to recognize if we are to understand the significance of later theories. This is the assumption that the character, the pattern, of an antibody was derived from the same pattern present in a group of body cells and deriving its special character presumably from genetic sources. A toxin was toxic because it had a structure that fitted in some complementary fashion to a genetically predetermined structure in the susceptible cell.

Since 1890 there has been a swelling flood of contributions on the things that happened when substances of all sorts were injected into experimental animals. It became evident that not only bacteria and bacterial poisons could produce antibodies. Serum or red blood cells from another animal species would serve almost equally well or even a purified protein like crystallized egg albumin. Finally in the 1930's Landsteiner found that by linking quite small chemical groups to protein he could produce artificial antigens which gave rise to antibody against the attached chemical groupings as well as against the carrier protein. This seemed to call for the abandonment of any idea that antibody patterns were preformed in the body before contact with the stimulating substance, by this time referred to as the *antigen*. Although it was subsequently modified by various authors, Landsteiner in 1937 put forward the basic view of antibody production which remained virtually unquestioned until 1956. He considered that when a foreign substance of the necessary physical and chemical qualities entered the body it was taken up by phagocytic cells and there served as a pattern or template against which globulin molecules could be synthesized. As a result the globulin was liberated, carrying two small areas on its surface which were exactly complementary to active patches or determinants of the antigen molecules that induced its production.

In the last year or two it has become the fashion to divide theories of immunity into selective theories and instructive theories, and it should be recognized at once that Ehrlich's and Landsteiner's theories exemplify the difference as well as any more modern formulations. In a *selective* theory it is assumed that the function of the antigen is to stimulate a pre-existent pattern into activity, in an *instructive* theory the antigen is assumed to impress a new pattern on the cell concerned.

Gradually cellular aspects of immunity began to extend beyond the rather nonspecific role of the phagocytes in dealing with invading bacteria. Probably the two most significant sets of phenomena were the tuberculin reaction and anaphylaxis in the guinea pig. If a man or a guinea pig is suffering from an infection with the tubercle bacillus and a small amount of a protein produced by the bacillus (tuberculin) is injected into his (or its) skin, a "delayed reaction" appears in the form of an area of redness and swelling not clearly visible until 18 or 24 hours after the injection. A number of other sorts of infection and a variety of chemical irritants can give essentially similar reactions. This phenomenon is referred to as delayed hypersensitivity and like the antibody reactions it is highly specific. A response to tuberculin indicates with certainty that the individual is, or has been, infected with tuberculosis. Quite another type of reagent will give a positive test (the Frei test) only in persons infected with viruses of the psittacosis-lymphogranuloma group.

Anaphylaxis in its classical form was discovered by Theobald Smith in the course of an attempt to be economical with guinea pigs and use survivors from one experiment for a second test. Most of his experiments were titrations of diphtheria antitoxin, which meant inoculating graded mixtures of toxin and antitoxin into the animals. Antitoxin is horse serum and it is characteristic of foreign serum proteins when injected into guinea pigs that they render the animal curiously vulnerable to a second injection. Theobald Smith found that some of these economy guinea pigs injected with horse serum or mixtures containing it collapsed and died within a minute or two, with symptoms resembling those of an acute asthmatic attack. The same sort of reaction with rather different symptoms can be seen in several other animal species, and in one form or another it is not uncommon in human beings. The essence of an anaphylactic reaction is that first contact with a foreign protein is harmless but subsequent injections may have harmful results because of a changed immunological situation within the body.

Both the tuberculin reaction and the anaphylactic response were obviously important for medicine, and both were soon found to be prototypes of a wide variety of phenomena, some of them to be seen in the clinic, others only in the laboratory. Though neither group is completely understood even yet, it gradually became clear that both were manifestations of the activity of *immunologically modified cells.* It had long been tacitly assumed that antibodies must be produced by cells, but otherwise the only cells of interest to the immunologist were the cells which could take in and digest bacteria, the microphages and macrophages of Metchnikoff. These new phenomena made biologists look much more closely at the significance of cells for the actual manifestations of immunity. Even more important was an indication that not all the manifestations of immunity were beneficial to the individual — that frank disease might even be produced by the body's "misguided" response to foreign material.

We might underline this by mentioning a simple fact. Since penicillin was introduced into medicine in 1941–42, it has saved many millions of lives but perhaps as many as a thousand people have died as a result of a hypersensitivity reaction following a second or later injection of penicillin. Although penicillin is not a protein, these penicillin reactions are basically similar to anaphylaxis.

The whole history of immunology has manifested a similar progressive broadening of interest beyond the starting concept of immunity to infection. As in the case of anaphylaxis, many of the advances resulted from the experimental analysis of mishaps. It was an obvious thought, once the nature of asepsis and the elementary rules of surgery had been grasped, that loss of blood in a patient might be made good by transfusion of blood from a healthy donor. Experience showed that, although about three-quarters of such transfusions were uneventful and often effective, far too many gave rise to serious illness. In 1904 Landsteiner found that human bloods could be divided into three (later four) groups and by about 1914 this knowledge began to be applied to make blood transfusion safe. But as experience of transfusion developed, it gradually became clear that no two bloods were quite the same and that very few patients who required repeated transfusions failed to develop some form of immunological response, not necessarily a dangerous one.

Even more disconcerting were the results of surgical attempts to replace a diseased or damaged organ by a similar tissue from a healthy donor or from a previously healthy victim of accidental death. There are some eventually fatal diseases of the kidney, for instance, in which replacement of the kidney by a healthy one, if it were possible, would almost certainly prolong the patient's life indefinitely. The body, however, will not accept foreign tissue. Within a few days the transplanted organ begins to cease functioning, inflammatory changes become evident, and if the patient survives the graft is completely rejected.

It is one of the concise statements of modern immunology that the body will accept as itself only what is genetically indistinguishable from the part replaced. It was an act of faith deserving of the success it achieved when a Boston surgeon sought out and found a few cases of gross kidney disease in patients who had an identical twin. In four out of six operations the results were successful; the healthy kidney was accepted, the surgical wounds healed, and the organ functioned effectively. It is as if the body can recognize its own individuality and will accept nothing that is inconsistent with that individuality.

Immunity against invading microorganisms is one manifestation of this imperative, but all recent developments in immunology suggest that immunity to infection is only a specialized aspect of a much wider and deeper topic. Immunology will probably always have a medical bias, but at the present time the growing edge of medical knowledge is concerned more with the anomalies of the immune process which produce disease than with the artificial development of immunity against infectious disease. Both aspects will be discussed extensively in this book, but essentially we are concerned with something more fundamental than either. Its aim is to discuss in language no more technical than is absolutely necessary the implications of the body's demand for the maintenance of its own integrity.

2. Antibodies

During one phase of the history of immunology, it was the tacit belief of most workers that all types of immunity were due to *antibodies*. These were thought of as chemical agents liberated into the blood, whose production had been provoked by substances (*antigens*), usually parts of microorganisms, which had entered the tissues in one way or another. Each antibody had an important role in preventing the harmful activities of the microorganism which provided the corresponding antigen. If this was true, it was obviously important to discover everything that could be discovered about antibodies and to summarize and coordinate that knowledge in an appropriate theoretical framework. Until very recently most theories of immunity have been theories on the nature and production of antibodies.

Antibodies are still of the greatest importance in medicine and in the control of animal disease. No understanding of immunology is possible without an adequate scrutiny of the facts of antibody production and of the physical and chemical nature of antibody itself. It is important, however, to grasp at once that the terms antibody and antibodies are very difficult to define, that immunity to disease is not wholly due to antibody, and that there are many aspects of immunology in which neither antibody nor immunity against microbial infection is involved.

In considering the significance of antibody, we can start with a child who is being immunized against diphtheria by a series of two or three injections of toxoid. This is a procedure which has been universally practiced in most advanced countries for 20 years or more. During that period diphtheria has diminished from a serious cause of death in childhood to something so rare that many medical students nowadays never see a case of the disease during their training. This is certainly not wholly due to immunization but the evidence is overwhelming that immunization played the major part.

Diphtheria is (or was) an infectious disease due to the lodging and multiplication of the diphtheria bacillus in the throat. The bacillus is not particularly invasive but it liberates an extremely poisonous substance, the diphtheria toxin, which kills adjacent cells and can have distant damaging effects on nerves and on the substance of the heart. Probably the most important action of the toxin is to damage and kill the cells in the immediate vicinity of the multiplying organisms. This provides a favorable niche of dead tissue for further multiplication and of course further production of toxin. As a result we have the production of the spreading gray membrane over the tonsil which is the characteristic sign of the disease.

The diphtheria bacillus was isolated in 1884 and a few years later it was shown that cultures of the organism contained a toxin, a poison that was quite distinct from the bacilli. The filtered fluid from the culture killed guinea pigs when a fraction of a milliliter was injected, and in very much smaller dose produced sharply defined areas of redness when injected superficially into the skin of rabbits or guinea pigs. In 1890 von Behring found that animals injected with nonfatal doses of toxin gradually became resistant to its action and developed in their serum something which could neutralize the killing power of the toxin. The substance responsible he called antitoxin.

At the time nothing was known of toxin and antitoxin beyond their functional activity. The broth culture contained something which in a certain dose regularly killed guinea pigs within 4 days. If a hundred times this amount of toxic broth was mixed with a milliliter of serum from an immunized horse, the mixture was harmless on injection into guinea pigs. By elaboration of tests like this it became possible to measure the relative strength of antitoxin in any sample of serum and so to determine whether it was suitable for the treatment of diphtheria. This was possible without any knowledge of the chemical nature of either agent.

The nature of toxin and antitoxin was gradually elucidated over the period 1890–1940; methods of treating and preventing diphtheria were discovered and refined and today most work on the problem is strictly routine. There are still gaps in our understanding of some of the basic phenomena, but from the practical angle the problems are solved.

The diphtheria toxin is chemically a simple protein built up only of amino acids. Its molecular weight is around 70,000, a very usual size for a protein. The pure material is extremely poisonous, 0.0001 mg being lethal for a guinea pig. Active work is going on about the possible ways by which diphtheria toxin exerts its action on the susceptible cell or animal. It now seems likely that the toxin interferes at some point in the process by which energy-producing substances are oxidized in the cell and that one or more of the iron-containing enzymes concerned in that process are affected. From the immunological point of view, however, the precise biochemical mechanism is not immediately important. All we are concerned with is that the toxin is a definable protein with a striking and measurable effect on experimental animals.

Antitoxin is readily available in the form of serum from an immunized horse and it can be accurately measured (titrated) against toxin. With modern biochemical techniques, it is nearly always possible to isolate from biological fluids or tissues any active agent in which the biochemist is interested so long as adequate raw material is available and there is a reasonably accurate method of measuring the biological activity in question. When isolated, antitoxin turned out to be exactly similar chemically to one of the normal protein components of the blood, gamma globulin. The only detectable difference between purified diphtheria antitoxin and gamma globulin obtained by the same procedure from a normal horse was that the former combined with the toxin, while the latter did not. This is the basic finding about all antibodies: they are normal globulin molecules with a subtle "pattern" difference, not yet expressible in chemical terms, which is responsible for their characteristic activity. By the modern techniques of physical chemistry, it has been found that "normal gamma globulin" is really a complex mixture of related proteins. The simple statement, therefore, requires some elaboration and qualification, as we shall see later. Essentially, however, it is still true and useful.

We can use the various interactions between diphtheria toxin and antitoxin to exemplify many of the practical and theoretical aspects of immunity. We might start with what happens in the test tube. Suppose we have a toxin and a serum from an immunized horse. If we mix equal amounts we shall quite probably find that the mixture becomes cloudy and within a few minutes develops a precipitate. If now we vary the proportions of toxin and serum in different mixtures, we can prepare a series of tubes, each containing the same amount of toxin but each having, say, 5 percent more antitoxin than the one preceding it. In such a series one tube will grow turbid and flocculate before any of the others. The proportions of the two reagents in this tube are just right to allow rapid union between them, and if we centrifuge out the precipitate, the clear supernatant fluid is found by appropriate tests to be free both of toxin and antitoxin. By suitable elaboration of such tests it can be shown that toxin and antitoxin combine unit for unit in essentially the same fashion as any other pair of chemical reagents. With modern refinements of technique that statement needs many qualifications, but this holds just as much for any other precipitation reaction involving very large molecules. The essential feature is that toxin-antitoxin union is basically no different from many other types of interaction between protein molecules.

With an active antitoxin and standard toxin, the point at which flocculation occurs is also at or very close to the neutral point where all toxicity is just neutralized. If with given reagents two volumes of toxin and one of serum give the optimal point of flocculation, we can be sure that if we dilute the toxin 1000 times and mix it with an equal volume of serum diluted 2000 times we shall have a neutral mixture. If 0.1 ml of this is injected into the skin of a rabbit or a man, there will be no more than a small pink spot, but if we halved the amount of serum the mixture would give a broad red area of inflammation. This is due to the damaging action of the unneutralized toxin on the skin cells.

This brings us to the Schick test, used to determine whether a child has been immunized naturally or artificially against diphtheria. Diphtheria toxin is diluted to such a degree that

0.1 ml contains one-fiftieth of the dose needed to kill a guinea pig. When this is injected into the skin of a person with no antitoxin in his blood, the red area of a positive Schick reaction is visible at the site within 24 hours. On the other hand, if the child has been immunized or has been mildly or invisibly infected naturally by the diphtheria bacillus, he will have a certain amount of antitoxin in his blood. If the amount is above a certain level (about 0.003 of an antitoxin unit), the antitoxin will neutralize the test dose of toxin before it can produce significant damage to local cells. In the days when first immunization against diphtheria was done in the schools, it was usual to immunize only those children with a positive Schick reaction, but with immunization in infancy now the universal practice the test is unnecessary as a routine.

The Schick test was the first example of a very important application of immunology to the understanding of infectious disease. In the days before immunization almost every child could be certain of being infected with the diphtheria bacillus at some time before his schooldays were over, but only a small minority of those infected developed recognizable symptoms. The others overcame the infection and in the process developed a measurable amount of antitoxin in their blood. At the same time, and more importantly, they gained resistance against exposure to a larger dose or a more virulent variety of the bacillus. These *subclinical* infections are of great importance in epidemiology. Frequently they are vastly more common than symptomatic infections, and unless their occurrence can be recognized it is quite impossible to understand the natural history of an infectious disease. The presence of the corresponding antibody in the blood is an almost infallible indication of the occurrence of infection in the past. If blood samples are taken from children at yearly intervals, the time at which infection occurred can be established. If a large number of children of different ages are tested at the same time, the proportion with antibody is found to increase with age and the characteristic pattern of that increase will often tell us a great deal about the disease. It is immaterial whether the antibody is recognized by tests on the serum or indirectly as in the Schick test. A negative Schick reaction has much the same significance as the measurement of 1/300 of a unit of antitoxin in the blood, and the test is very much simpler to do.

Everyone knows that immunization against diphtheria is done by injecting a harmless derivative of the toxin produced by treating it with dilute formalin. From our present point of view, toxoid, as the nontoxic derivative is called, is important because of its indication that only parts of an antigenic molecule are necessary for the production of immunity. Toxoid is harmless, but in all its reactions with antitoxin it behaves precisely like toxin and it has the same capacity to stimulate antitoxin production.

Everything that has been said so far would indicate that the interaction of diphtheria toxin and antitoxin was as regular as the neutralization of an acid by an alkali. This is, in fact, far from being the case. We can pass over the common occurrence of "nonavid" antitoxin which gives anomalous results in the standard tests because of a looser type of union between the reagents. A more interesting example was observed by Kuhns and Pappenheimer in New York when they were testing pure toxoid as an immunizing agent on a group of medical students. Most of the students reacted normally, but a few responded to the injection as if it had been a grass-pollen extract in a sufferer from hay fever. These abnormal people, in fact, all suffered from one allergic condition or another. If serum is obtained from one of these individuals after the immunization has been completed, it can be shown to

contain antitoxin. When the standard test is made by injecting mixtures of toxin and serum into the skin of a rabbit, good
neutralization is evident. In the test tube, however, no cloud-
ing or flocculation occurred with any of the mixtures, not
even in those which from the neutralization test should have
been the "right" mixtures. These allergic subjects ran true
to form when tested by a small injection of toxoid into the
skin — quite harmless in normal individuals. Their response
was to give the "wheal and flare" reaction known to any hay-
fever patient who has ever been tested by an allergist.

It is important to realize that antibodies may differ among
themselves even when prepared in the same species against
the same antigen. The specific pattern that allows an antibody to unite with its corresponding antigen may be built
into more than one type of soluble protein and, as we shall
see, it may also be attached in some fashion to the surface of
certain cells.

Antibodies can be directed against bacteria as such as well
as against the toxins they produce. When a man recovers from
an attack of bacillary dysentery, it will be found with great
regularity that his serum will cause a visible change in a culture of the strain of dysentery bacillus responsible for the
attack. With normal serum the culture remains uniformly
turbid but with the patient's serum the bacilli in the culture
stick together when they collide and gradually agglutinate
into easily visible clumps which settle to the bottom of the
tube. This is the agglutination reaction, which is used not only
to recognize the existence of past infection but also to classify
bacterial strains into species and subspecies.

The action of the antibody here is to unite with the antigenic patterns on the surface of the bacteria or on the con-
tractile threads — flagella — that are responsible for the mobil-
ity of some bacteria. Most immunochemists believe that an

antibody molecule has usually two active groups, so that a single molecule can, in principle, serve to bind two bacteria together. A clump of agglutinated bacteria on this view is a crude lattice in which bacteria are held together by molecular bridges of antibody. Others are dubious of the lattice theory and think that the main effect of the attachment of antibody is to replace part of the bacterial surface with denatured gamma globulin. This so modifies the physical nature of the surface that it has a lower electric charge and the bacteria are then "precipitated" if the salt concentration in the suspending fluid is appropriate.

We are not specially interested here in how the dysentery bacilli cause disease, or how the bacteriologist classifies them into species and serological types. Nevertheless dysentery is a very important disease, and a great deal of work on the agglutination of dysentery bacilli by serum from patients or from specially immunized rabbits is always going on. If we are doing this sort of work and have an interest a little wider than the immediate significance of the tests, we shall come across results of great importance for immunological theory.

Suppose we have a dozen distinct cultures of dysentery bacilli which have previously been shown to be related by the fact that all are to some degree agglutinated by a certain immune serum. We want to determine how many types of bacteria there are in the group. To do so we would probably start by immunizing rabbits against each of the strains which had been chosen for any reason as possible prototypes of different groups. For the sake of simplicity we can concentrate on a single serum made against strain A. The serum agglutinates a standard suspension of bacillus A very strongly. Its strength can be estimated by finding the degree to which it can be diluted before it just fails to cause agglutination. If this dilution is 1 in 10,000, it is conventional to say that the titer of the serum is 10,000. It would be more in line with normal scientific procedure to determine how much antibody globulin was needed to produce nearly complete agglutination and express the strength of the serum in terms of so many milligrams of antibody per liter. But, for reasons which will emerge, it is quite possible that this might give only a deceptive appearance of accuracy and that the rough and ready method is the most practical one. If we test the same serum against strains B, C, D, and E, we shall find that they also are agglutinated but not so strongly. When a bacterium is agglutinated it attaches antibody to itself and, as it were, precipitates out of solution that fraction of antibody which will combine with it. If then we keep on adding strain B to a given amount of serum, a point will be reached when all the antibody is precipitated. We now get rid of all the bacteria by centrifuging or filtering the mixture and test this *absorbed* serum on our whole series. It agglutinates B not at all but its activity against A is unaltered. In Table 1 are shown the sort of results that would be obtained if we absorbed serum A with each of the strains separately and with all the strains except A.

It will be noticed that A removes all antibody, that B is equivalent to E, and that all cross reactions can be removed while still leaving activity against the strain used for immunization only slightly reduced. One look at the table tells us at once that antibody against A is not a single substance, "antibody A." It is clearly composed of a *population* of molecules which have one feature in common, ability to react and unite with components on the surface of A bacteria. The different elements of the population differ widely in their capacity to react with different but related strains. This quality allows us to prepare from the rather nondescript original serum a highly specific reagent, like that on the bottom row which

Table 1. *Cross reaction and absorption of an antiserum.*

Serum A	Titer against —				
	A	B	C	D	E
Unabs.	10,000	500	5,000	2,000	400
Abs. A	0	0	0	0	0
Abs. B	10,000	0	5,000	2,000	0
Abs. C	8,000	200	0	500	200
Abs. D	10,000	0	1,000	0	0
Abs. E	10,000	0	5,000	2,000	0
Abs. B,C, D, E	5,000	0	0	0	0

will agglutinate only strains that are virtually identical with A.

Exactly the same sort of results will be obtained if we use related influenza viruses as antigens, or, for the matter of that, two related pure crystalline proteins, such as hen-egg albumin and duck-egg albumin. There is no exception to the rule that an antiserum is a heterogeneous population of molecules.

There are even differences among antibody molecules when we examine them simply from the standpoint of physical chemistry. Blood serum is a very complex mixture of proteins with smaller amounts of salts and with traces of almost every significant biochemical substance to be found in the body. The serum proteins can be separated into groups by various physical processes, the most commonly used being electrophoresis. Essentially, this is the application of an electric current to separate substances which move faster in an electric field from those which move more slowly. By a suitable technique we can make a sample of serum draw a graph of its own constitution (Fig. 1). All but traces of antibody are found in the gamma globulin fraction and it is a useful approximation to the truth to say that all antibodies are composed of gamma globulin. Many workers in immunity speculate that all gamma globulin is probably antibody of one sort or another.

Much more refined methods of isolating proteins have been developed in recent years. Perhaps it is more in line with present thought to say that more and more powerful methods

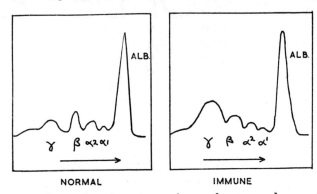

NORMAL   IMMUNE

Fig. 1. Electrophoretic patterns of normal serum and serum from a person producing large amounts of antibody. The peaks represent protein components moving with different velocities in an electric field. Albumin (ALB) is the fastest-moving and most abundant component. Then follow the globulins, labeled in order α_1, α_2, β, and γ. Antibody is found predominantly in the γ peak.

are becoming available for dividing heterogeneous populations of protein molecules into subpopulations, each with a much narrower range of variability. Only with some highly specialized proteins like insulin is it possible to obtain anything one could call a pure protein, that is, a uniform population of molecules. Using chromatographic techniques it is possible to split "gamma globulin" into several fractions, and often more than one fraction will include a proportion of antibody.

Proteins can also be separated by sufficiently powerful centrifugal forces. In human serum, gamma globulin is found to contain two main components, a light one with a molecular weight about 160,000 and a heavy component with a molecular weight near to 1,000,000. Some antibodies fall in one set, some in the other.

These physical characters of antibody are of great practical importance in providing ways of preparing highly concentrated antibody free of all the unnecessary and potentially harmful components also present in crude antiserum. From the point of view of those mainly interested in the biological side of immunity, the physical and chemical qualities of antibodies are not particularly important. Biochemists have, however, tended to dominate thought and experiment in immunology for many years and they have naturally pressed the chemical study of antibody to the limit. It will be convenient at this stage, however, to leave any further discussion of the chemical side until we deal with the theories of immunity, particularly with the characteristically chemical approach of Pauling's "instructive" theory of antibody production.

As our final example of antibody in relation to infection, we can take the antibody against polio virus that appears after an attack of paralytic polio or after immunization with the Salk vaccine. The normal way in which such antibody is detected and measured is by a neutralization test. A known amount of virus is mixed with graded amounts of antiserum and each mixture is tested for unneutralized virus. Ten years ago this would have meant injecting each into the brains of monkeys and watching for paralysis. Since tissue-culture methods were developed in the early 1950's, the mixtures have been inoculated into tissue cultures prepared from monkey kidney cells. If there is still active virus present, it will infect the cells and within a few days produce easily visible damage. If the antibody has been effective, the cells show no differences from uninoculated control cultures.

With appropriate technical methods it is a routine matter

to determine for any specimen of serum whether there is antibody against the three immunological types of polio virus and how much against each. Basically, polio antibody is quite similar to those we have mentioned earlier. It is a serum protein, a gamma globulin, which can unite with the surface of the virus particle and by so doing render it noninfective. Just how this takes place we do not know, but this ignorance of the actual process of neutralization is no bar to an operationally effective understanding of the practical aspects of immunity to poliomyelitis.

In broad terms, antibody in the blood, whether it is put there in the form of gamma globulin produced by others or has been actively produced in response to Salk immunization, protects against polio because its presence provides a block in the pathway which the virus must take to reach the spinal cord. Polio virus enters the body through the bowel in most instances and, after a preliminary phase of multiplication in the intestinal wall, seeps through into the blood. From the blood it is able in a small unfortunate minority of children to penetrate into the susceptible areas of the spinal cord. If the virus is regularly inactivated by antibody as soon as it enters the blood, there can be no possibility of its invading the nervous system. The virus may multiply freely in the intestinal wall but as far as the child's health is concerned this is of no importance.

Salk vaccine is prepared from polio virus grown in tissue culture and killed with formalin under such conditions that the significant antigenic patterns of the virus are unchanged. For technical reasons the actual amount of virus protein in the usual dose is very small and in order to obtain a satisfactory production of antibody at least three injections are necessary. A long interval of 6–8 months is advised between the second and third injections. With potent vaccine the standard three-shot course produces antibody in the child's blood to the same sort of level that one would expect to find after a natural attack of paralytic disease, and considerably higher than after a much commoner subclinical attack. Experience indicates that such a level of antibody will provide absolute protection against natural infection and paralysis with the corresponding types of virus.

There is no doubt about the safety and effectiveness of properly prepared Salk vaccine, but there are certain difficulties in being sure that it has been prepared at full potency. The search for a better method of immunization has in recent years led to the development of a "living attenuated" vaccine; but the principles involved here could be more satisfactorily considered at a later stage. There is very much more that could be said about antibodies, and in particular it should be stressed that there are antibodies that have other activities than protection against this or that infectious disease. So far we have been concerned with antibody against a clearly definable agent coming from outside the body: a bacterium, a virus, or a toxin. The activity of the antibody in protecting against the harmful agent could be used to define and measure it. But the total immunological situation is a more subtle one. There are globulins in animal serum which behave precisely like antibodies in their reactions with certain substances but have certainly not been produced by any conventional type of immunization. The simplest examples are concerned with the human blood groups, and in the next chapter these are discussed in relation to other aspects of immunological individuality.

3. Blood Groups and Natural Antibodies

From the earliest times it must have seemed reasonable that the effects of hemorrhage might be remedied by the transfusion of blood from a healthy donor. There were, of course, completely insuperable practical difficulties, from clotting and from bacterial contamination, which blocked the effective use of blood until the development of modern medical science, but the possibilities of transfusion had been actively discussed in scientific circles since the earliest days of the Royal Society. With the development of simple anticoagulants like sodium citrate and the technique of aseptic surgery and sterile handling of fluids, blood transfusion became practicable and in many cases was highly successful. We know today that if blood is taken at random from one person and given to another without any form of "cross typing," in about 75 percent of instances no harm will be done. With the other combinations, however, serious and even fatal reactions might ensue.

In 1904 Landsteiner described how serum from some persons clumped the red cells of some others and showed how there was a simple set of rules for predicting the results of mixing different cells and serums. Slightly modified, his formulation was as follows. Human beings can be divided into four groups, AB, A, B, and O, according to whether their blood cells are agglutinated by both anti-A and anti-B serum, by anti-A alone, by anti-B alone, or by neither. In every individual the serum contains all those antibodies which will not agglutinate (clump) the person's own cells. For our four types, then, the red cells and serum antibodies — the so-called isoagglutinins — can be tabulated as in Table 2.

Table 2. The human ABO blood groups.

Antigens on red cells	AB	A	B	O
Isoagglutinins in serum	Nil	anti-B	anti-A	anti-A, anti-B

This is a beautifully simple arrangement, but even as it stands it has some quite abstruse implications. It made it possible to use blood transfusion safely, but it is also fair to say that ever since Landsteiner hematologists have been finding more and more different ways by which difficulties can arise from putting blood from one person into another.

Sometimes Nature herself creates difficulties of this sort: the Rh baby, for instance. The present interpretation of Rh blood groups is too complex to attempt a complete account here. It is legitimate, however, to concentrate on the most important aspect and speak simply of Rh-positive and Rh-negative individuals. The difference is genetic in origin and is dependent on the presence or absence of the genes D and d in one of the chromosomes. Closely associated are two other allelic pairs, Cc and Ee, but these are not often responsible for trouble and we shall say no more about them.

If the gene D is present either as DD or Dd, the person is Rh-positive; in its absence, that is with the genetic composition dd, the person is Rh-negative. The gene D controls the appearance of an antigenic pattern on the cells, which can be called either D or Rh+. This is a "good" antigen; that is, when Rh+ cells are injected into an Rh-negative person, the latter is very likely to develop an anti-Rh antibody. Theoretically, the antigen corresponding to dd might produce antibody in a person with the genetic make-up DD, but this is an excessively rare occurrence.

The D antigen becomes very important in medicine because of the possibility of serious or fatal disease in the offspring of Rh+ fathers and Rh− mothers. A high proportion of the offspring will be Rh+, 100 percent if the father is DD, 50 percent if he is Dd. During the course of pregnancy some leakage occurs across the normal barrier in the placenta that separates the mother's circulation from the baby's. There is no doubt that, when immunologically mature lymphoid (white) cells of the mother are stimulated by red cells of the embryo which are different from those of the mother, antibodies can be produced.

If the mother is Rh− her cells can produce antibody if they are stimulated by the antigen D (Rh+). This undoubtedly occurs in the condition called hemolytic disease of the newborn, and the usual interpretation is that cells from the embryo leak into the maternal circulation and in the mother stimulate her tissues to produce antibody. This passes across the placenta in the way all antibodies do and produces massive damage to the baby's red cells in the period immediately after birth. Quite recently the possibility has been mooted that very similar conditions might be produced if some of the mother's leukocytes could leak into the fetal circulation, implant in spleen and bone marrow, and there produce the damaging antibody. There is as yet no proof that this has occurred but, as will be mentioned later, there are some good experimental precedents. For the present we can adopt the standard interpretation that "Rh disease" is due to antibody produced by the mother in response to the stimulus of the red cells of her genetically different fetus.

Hemolytic disease of the newborn was recognized as an immunological disease only in 1940–41. Since then many thousands of cases have been studied and a great many other types of immunological malfunctioning recognized. In modern life there are three ways only by which blood cells, white or red, can find themselves in the circulation of another individual. The first is in the course of pregnancy as has been described; the second is by therapeutic transfusion of blood; and, for completeness, the third is through fusion of the placental circulation to two nonidentical twins so that they have a common pool of circulating cells. The anomalies following repeated pregnancies or repeated transfusions have provided a rich fund of material for investigation and thrown new light on the complexity of human make-up.

We can summarize the position as follows. In human beings there is first the ABO system of blood groups by which people can be divided into four groups, the proportions of which vary according to race but in Western Europeans are about 4 percent AB, 47 percent A, 6 percent B, and 43 percent O. In each group there is also present in the serum agglutinin (natural antibody) against all those types of antigen not carried by the cells. In addition there are large numbers of differences in immunological pattern which are potentially capable of being brought to light by the mixing of bloods which may result either from pregnancy or from transfusion. These differences can be arranged in relation to a number of blood-group systems, each of which can be regarded as associated with a cluster of linked or alternative genes at a certain locus on one chromosome. In most of these systems we have a division into types each of which is represented by a substantial proportion of people; for example, in the simplest form of Rh grouping there are 17 percent of dd, 48 percent of Dd, and 35 percent of DD in European populations. There are ten blood-group systems of this sort that have been described, plus a number of so-called private blood groups in which only a single family appears to differ from the rest of humanity.

There are some important biological implications arising from this work on human blood groups; the first is the genetic polymorphism of the human species. To the geneticist this immediately presents a problem of origins. Why and how, for instance, did Asian races in general come to have a much higher proportion of group B individuals than is found among Western Europeans?

It was natural to look for some indication that the nature of his blood group might in one way or another influence the survival of the individual. Two sorts of investigation have given results. It has been found that persons of group O are more prone than others to duodenal ulcer and those of group A to gastric ulcer and gastric cancer. There may be one or two other associations of the same type. An entirely different sort of investigation has shown that when parents differ in their blood groups there is an increased likelihood that the child will die before or immediately after birth. The likelihood is very small in any given case but the result can be seen in any large-scale study of blood-group statistics. It is clear, therefore, that there are ways by which selective survival might operate in relation to blood groups.

Another very important factor is genetic drift, the change in average genetic character that can result when a small fraction of a former population, a single family, say, gives rise eventually to a new population. In the early stages of man's spread across the continents, there were probably quite frequent occasions when a single family group might be the sole originators of a substantial population. For one reason or another different races now differ widely in the proportions of each blood group in the population, and data on blood-group distribution are now almost the most important requirement of the physical anthropologist. The study of blood groups has in fact probably contributed as much to anthropology and the history and prehistory of human migration and mixings as it has to medicine and immunology.

We are not concerned here with the anthropological implications of the blood groups, but we are deeply interested in that other implication that can be summarized in Medawar's phrase, the uniqueness of the individual.

The red cells of the blood have no nucleus and are much simpler in their construction than any other cells of the body. Even so, we now know of more than 50 different immunological qualities whose presence or absence on the red cell can be tested for in any sample of human blood. The chance that any two individuals (not identical twins) will be the same in all these respects is negligibly small. Each of these immunological differences depends on relatively small chemical patterns on one of the types of protein or polysaccharide molecules that help to build up the red-cell surface. A given type of red cell can act as an antigen and provoke the appearance of antibody only when it is introduced into the circulation of someone who does *not* possess that type of red cell, but even under such circumstances antibody may not be produced.

Blood groups have all been worked out from responses occurring in human beings and we can be sure that, in addition to the chemical configurations we have been discussing, there must be at least an equal number which could be antigenic patterns were they not common to all human beings. The problem of why a chemical pattern is not antigenic in any animal which possesses that pattern as part of its bodily structure is probably the most important of all immunological questions. Fifty years' experience of blood transfusion, with its difficulties and catastrophes and the efforts to understand and overcome them, has taught immunologists a great deal. Probably more than anything else it has been responsible for defining this central problem of the differentiation between self and not-self.

The third aspect of blood-group experience that has wide general significance is usually referred to as the difference between a primary and a secondary immune response. It is the almost invariable experience to find that a child with severe Rh disease is the third or later in the family. First entry of Rh-positive cells into the mother's body does not provoke any significant amount of antibody. Its effect is to sensitize the body to react more extensively and dangerously to renewed contact with the same antigenic pattern. It seems that first contact sets in process something equivalent to tooling up in a factory. Only when this is complete can effective production begin.

Pediatric experience of hemolytic disease of the newborn has probably provided the most dramatic example of this difference between primary and secondary response but there are many others which come within common experience. The general practice of having the third and final shot of a Salk vaccine course 6 to 7 months after the second is to allow the full development of the potentialities of the secondary response. If a man suffers a compound fracture liable to be contaminated with tetanus bacilli, it is standard practice to give him an injection of tetanus toxoid if it is *known* that he had been previously immunized. This will give him a secondary response in time to have much antitoxin in circulation before any toxin produced in the wound can build up to a dangerous level (Fig. 2). In a similar case where the patient has not

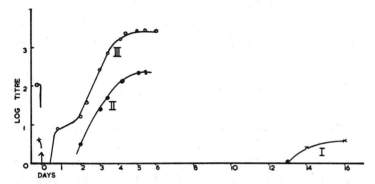

FIG. 2. To show the difference between primary and secondary responses. A rabbit was immunized by three injections of staphylococcal toxoid by the intravenous route. The antitoxic responses are shown: I, small and delayed; II and III, given 3 and 26 weeks later, show rapid and high-level responses.

been immunized, the primary response to toxoid would be too slow to be effective and he would have to be given ready-made antitoxin — the ATS (antitetanic serum) of the casualty ward.

There are very few aspects of immunology which cannot be exemplified by human experience with blood groups and the like. Take, for instance, the case of the young woman who was found with nearly half her red blood cells "really" belonging to her twin brother who had died as an infant. Mrs. McK. was a healthy volunteer blood donor, whose blood on routine testing with an anti-A serum showed clumps of agglutinated A cells among a lot of quite unagglutinated cells. It was soon established that she had, in fact, two sorts of cells, 61 percent of group O and 39 percent of group A. There were two other group differences in addition and from the status of the woman as a "secretor" of O substance it is clear that the 61 percent of O cells are hers but the 39 percent of A cells are genetically her brother's. There are also two pairs of living twins who are known to have shared their blood cells in this same fashion and the phenomenon is regularly seen in cattle twins.

The occurrence of two genetically distinct types of cell in one individual constitutes him a chimera, and much study has recently been directed toward understanding the conditions under which chimeras can be produced. Confining ourselves for the present to Nature's own experiments, the requirements are that the twins should be genetically dissimilar, that is, derived from two separately fertilized ova, and that their circulation makes use of a common part of the placenta so that blood cells and the cells from which blood cells spring can pass freely from one twin to the other.

Under these conditions we find that the wrong cells can become comfortably implanted in their foreign host, although we can be quite certain that if such cells were introduced after birth they would be rejected and would provoke an antibody response of the same general character as we have described in connection with hemolytic disease of the newborn. Implantation in embryonic life, then, has allowed the body to develop a tolerance of the foreign cells. Many other examples of this phenomenon have been described and it is referred to as *specific immunological tolerance*.

In the case of Mrs. McK., who was genetically of blood group O, one would have expected that her serum would contain anti-A and anti-B antibodies. If, however, she had had anti-A this would have reacted with and probably eliminated the circulating A cells. In fact, there was no trace of anti-A agglutinin in her serum, and appropriate tests made it certain that she was not producing and probably had never produced the antibody.

Here we see again the principle that the healthy body will never react immunologically against its own constituents. If a foreign cell or (with some limitations) a foreign protein is presented to the body during embryonic life and for one reason or another retained there well into adult life, it is accepted as part of the self and in some fashion an inhibition, a taboo, is established which ensures that it is immunologically respected just as rigidly as the genetically appropriate components of the body.

There are good evolutionary reasons why this should be so but it has proved very difficult to understand the machinery by which what may be called the recognition of self and not-self is achieved. In none of the earlier theories of immunity is any attempt made to cover this feature, though all have admitted its importance. Ehrlich spoke of a "horror autotoxicus," an expression that has much in common with the old dogma that nature abhors a vacuum.

As a preliminary to later discussion of the theories of immunity, it may be wise to speculate a little about the evolutionary significance of this matter of the recognition of foreignness. There will be more to be said about immunological tolerance in relation to cells and transplanted tissue in Chapter 6, but at this stage we should consider the simpler problem of how microorganismal invaders can be recognized as something alien and inappropriate to the body.

It may be felt intuitively that no explanation is really needed. Surely it is axiomatic that a virus getting into the body and damaging cells will automatically be recognized as something foreign and inimical. But it is not axiomatic. There is a virus disease of mice, lymphocytic choriomeningitis, in which large amounts of virus may be present in the body without provoking any detectable production of antibody and, it may be added, without producing signs of disease.

We are, in fact, concerned with two sorts of recognition. In the first place a microorganism never previously encountered must be recognized as foreign in order to allow the initiation of effective defense measures against it. After recovery, if the patient is to be immune, his cells must be able to recognize the pattern of the microorganism as something pertaining individually to an invader they have met and overcome in the past. The difference between the instructive and the selective approaches to immunity can again be mentioned in relation to these two types of recognition. The selective theories believe that both types of recognition are qualitatively similar; the immune recognition is far more effective merely because of the much larger number of cells and antibody molecules that are involved. Any instructive theory, on the other hand, must hold that the first recognition is by some means quite distinct from the second (immune) type. Some authorities would probably deny that primary recognition as alien is needed at all. The only type of recognition that is significant for them is assumed to be impressed on cells which take in the foreign substance or organism and functions only in relation to later contacts with the antigen.

If we provisionally accept a selection-type approach as that more susceptible to an evolutionary interpretation, we must regard the evolution of immunity as a complex process that at every stage would need to be coordinated with the development of other bodily faculties. We can picture three major capacities that must have evolved in step with each other:

1. The capacity of the organism to maintain its bodily form and dynamic equilibrium, involving not only the spatial relations between cells but their metabolic interactions one on the other; this must incidentally involve some means of "recogniz-

ing" when these relations are upset or menaced and of initiating corrective action;

2. The capacity to recognize as foreign any invading microorganism that has entered the tissues, and to use this as a trigger initiating defensive action;

3. The ability to develop, as a result of experience of a given antigen (organism or foreign macromolecule), a qualitatively and quantitatively heightened ability to react with the agent that has been met and overcome.

If there is a true primary ability to recognize a virus or bacterium as foreign, there are only two basic mechanisms that need to be considered. Either body cells and their products carry adequate "information" to allow them to recognize that the pattern on the invader is of a type positively recorded in that "library" of information as "foreign"; or the foreign surface has some quality that could not be present in any body component, such as groupings which are insusceptible to any body enzyme or a configuration that would bind gamma globulin by other than its immunologically reactive patches.

The difficulty of deciding between these alternatives for any given pathogenic microorganism is one of the best reasons for concentrating on antigens (cellular or soluble) derived from vertebrate sources in any experimental or theoretical approach to the problem of differentiation between self and notself.

4. Immune Reactions Not Related to Antibody

So far we have been wholly concerned with antibodies, the soluble proteins in the blood which can attach specifically to the corresponding antigens, producing various detectable and measurable results in the test tube or in the experimental animal. It is current and probably correct teaching that immunity against a second attack of infectious disease is mediated primarily by antibodies. There are, however, a variety of phenomena which have all the quality of immunological reactions in which antibody plays no part. Perhaps the most impressive example is seen in certain children who are born with a genetic inability to produce gamma globulin and antibody. As might be expected, such children are highly susceptible to pneumonia, and until a few years ago all of them must have died in infancy. Now, however, careful use of antibiotics and of normal human serum will usually allow them to maintain fair health. They have no detectable antibodies of any sort in their serum and a priori one would have thought that this would be a crippling weakness against virus diseases like measles. It was, therefore, something of a shock to find that children with this condition of *agammaglobulinemia* could pass through a typical attack of measles, recover normally, and show the normal continuing resistance to reinfection. Most would also respond normally to vaccination against smallpox. Clearly there are ways of developing immunity which do not depend on antibodies.

Long before agammaglobulinemia was recognized it was known that the tuberculin reaction first developed by Koch was also in some sense an immune reaction without benefit of antibodies. This is the prototype of what is now called delayed hypersensitivity, a process of great importance for the understanding of immunity.

Koch found that the tubercle bacillus in the course of its growth liberated a characteristic protein into the culture fluid. This, when separated from living and dead tubercle bacilli and concentrated, was called tuberculin. If a small amount of tuberculin was injected into the skin of a healthy guinea pig nothing happened. There was no temperature rise and no change at the site of injection. If, on the other hand, a guinea pig in which a tuberculous infection of the lymph glands had been induced a few weeks previously was given a similar injection, there ensued a violent local and general reaction. Twenty-four hours after the injection the local skin was hot, red, and thickened, and the body temperature was well above normal. With properly adjusted doses similar results obtain in human beings. If we inject a standard dose of tuberculin — now a much purer preparation than those used by Koch — into the skin of a person who has never been infected with the tubercle bacillus, there is no reaction. If, however, the individual is tuberculous or has recovered from even a symptomless infection with the tubercle bacillus, he will give a positive Mantoux or tuberculin test. Around the site of inoculation a red area will slowly develop, well marked at 24 hours and about its maximum in 48 hours.

The tuberculin test is specific and indicates that the body has been appropriately stimulated or sensitized by products of the tubercle bacillus, usually as a result of natural infection. Immunization with the living attenuated tubercle bacillus BCG will also produce a positive reaction. These are the only two circumstances that need be considered when we see a person with a positive tuberculin test. This specificity points strongly toward an immunological reaction, but in the past this conclusion was resisted because no corresponding antibody was present in persons or animals giving a tuberculin reaction. It was known that there were some types of skin reaction which could be shown to depend on the presence of an antibody in the blood. Many people have had experience of the allergist's skin tests to determine which type of pollen is causing their hay fever. If a person is sensitive to rye-grass pollen, injection of an extract of this pollen into his skin will rapidly induce the appearance of an itchy wheal surrounded by a bright red flare. It is immaterial what part of the skin is used for such a test, and one must assume that in some way the sensitization has been spread around the body by the blood. Evidence that antibody is responsible for this reaction comes from the fact that experimentally one can transfer this type of reactivity to a normal person by using serum from the patient's blood. About 1 ml of serum from A, the susceptible individual, is injected carefully to infiltrate a marked square inch of skin in B, the normal subject. Next day B is tested with the pollen extract to which A is sensitive. In the marked area he shows the same raised and itchy reaction as A but nothing on any distant area of skin. This transfer by serum, by antibody, fails completely with the tuberculin reaction, in guinea pigs or in men. But the susceptibility can be transferred from one guinea pig to another if we use cells of the lymph glands or spleen. It is now known that the tuberculin reaction is the prototype of a whole series of immunological responses which develop only under circumstances more or less analogous to those associated with a chronic infection. The agents which react with the antigen (tuberculin or some equivalent) are cells, almost certainly lymphocytes and monocytes (see Chapter 5), and no antibody is concerned. The interpretation that is favored by most immunologists is that in one way or another a population of reactive lymphocytes, "immunologically competent cells," appears in the body and circulates among many more cells of like appearance but without their specific reactivity. When a cell makes contact with the antigen with which it is keyed to react, a trigger is pulled and the cell suffers a little internal explosion. That is an attempt to express what occurs in metaphorical terms which tell almost as much as any other summary of the facts. All we know is that in the vicinity of a source of antigen lymphocytes and similar cells accumulate and products of cell damage produce a variety of disturbances of the capillary circulation that we see as a red patch.

These delayed-hypersensitivity reactions are basically indications of the presence of immunologically competent cells which must undoubtedly play an important part in defense against infection. It is highly significant that children with agammaglobulinemia who are incapable of producing antibody can nevertheless develop a variety of reactions of this delayed-hypersensitivity type. In all probability this is the most basic aspect of immunity, the development of cell populations which in the first instance can react directly with the antigen and at a later stage give rise to other cells capable of actually making antibody. Both types of cells are included under the term immunologically competent cells. In all attempts to understand immunology it is very important to consider these cellular aspects as well as the production of the classical antibody against toxins, viruses, and bacteria.

In Chapter 2 we described the two sorts of antibody which could be produced in response either to natural immunization by the diphtheria bacillus or by artificial immunization with diphtheria toxoid. Toxoid is a bland protein which is made by treating toxin with formalin so as to destroy its poisonous quality without modifying its antigenicity. It can be isolated in pure form and as such can be used to induce a state of delayed hypersensitivity analogous to the tuberculin reaction. To produce such a state in a guinea pig, toxoid-antitoxin precipitate is prepared from a flocculation reaction between purified toxoid and antitoxin prepared in a rabbit. The precipitate is suspended in fluid and a very small amount is injected into the guinea pig's skin.

Within a few days the guinea pig becomes extremely sensitive to an injection of a minute amount of toxoid into the skin, giving the typical slowly appearing red patch, but has no antibody in the blood. The situation is a delicately balanced one, however. It is only necessary to give another moderately sized dose of toxoid to provoke antibody production and to eliminate the hypersensitivity of the skin. This "desensitization" is mainly due to the presence of antibody in the blood and tissue fluids. Most of the toxoid injected in a skin test will combine with antibody and so have no capacity to trigger off any immunologically competent cells entering the adjacent tissues. The team of immunologists led by Pappenheimer at New York University holds that the first step in all immune reactions is the appearance of this cellular reactivity which is manifested by the delayed-hypersensitivity response. Most other authorities would probably agree in general but would raise the possibility that perhaps these cells had been made reactive by taking up small amounts of antibody.

This transfer of reactivity or sensitization of cells by antibody undoubtedly occurs under certain circumstances. In Chapter 1, Theobald Smith's discovery of anaphylaxis in guinea pigs was described but only typical active anaphylaxis was mentioned. A guinea pig treated weeks or months previously with horse serum is given a dose of the same foreign protein into the circulation and dies within 4 minutes from contraction of the bronchial muscles — virtually a lethal form of asthma. But the same symptoms can be induced in quite a different fashion. We immunize a guinea pig or a rabbit with the foreign protein until there is plenty of precipitating antibody in its serum. One or two milliliters of this serum is then injected into the test guinea pig. Twenty-four hours is allowed for the antibody to become attached to cells and then the guinea pig is "challenged" with a suitable dose of the foreign protein. If all the technical procedures have been correctly followed, this "passively sensitized" guinea pig will die with the same symptoms as the actively sensitized one. Analysis of this reaction many years ago by Sir Henry Dale showed that it resulted essentially from attachment of antibody to cells in various parts of the body and that this attachment provided a trigger which when it was activated by contact with antigen caused the cell to release histamine and possibly other substances. The symptoms of anaphylaxis were due to the local and general action of the histamine liberated. An injection of histamine will in fact produce almost exactly the same fatal symptoms as anaphylactic shock.

It is not within the scope of this book to go deeply into chemical and pharmacological aspects but a little should be said here, as it were in parentheses, of the "pharmacologically active substances" that cells liberate on damage. It is a commonplace that when skin is burnt or scalded, or a local boil develops, inflammation soon supervenes and we have the classical symptoms of "rubor, turgor, calor, dolor," that is, redness, swelling, heat, and pain. These symptoms are associated with dilatation of the small blood vessels, slowing of blood flow, increased exudation of fluid through the capillary walls and various cellular changes. All of these can be ascribed to the liberation of products of cell damage. From the nature of things a severely damaged cell must liberate a vast medley of substances, and the progress of research has led to a concentration on what is liberated from very lightly damaged cells and on cells which respond to what might be called physiological damage. There is a group of cells, the mast cells, found in many tissues which on gentle stimulation liberate heparin, histamine, and 5-hydroxytryptamine. Many types of cell liberate an enzyme with the physical character of a globulin which is extremely potent as an agent for producing inflammation in the guinea pig. Several other agents have been described but these are the only ones which need to be discussed — and then only briefly.

Histamine is a derivative of the amino acid histidine by decarboxylation. It undoubtedly plays a part in the normal economy of the body but no one has provided a simple account of what that normal function is. It is of great importance in allergic states of all sorts, and a whole series of drugs, the antihistamines, have found a big market for the treatment of hay fever and asthma. 5-hydroxytryptamine (serotonin) is a somewhat similar derivative of the amino acid tryptophan, with its main action on the vascular system and of more importance in mice and rats than in other animals. Heparin is a complex polysaccharide which is the only body component that has a strong action in preventing the clotting of normal blood. Little more need be said about the inflammatory globulin but we should mention that there is good evidence that products from damaged cells can (*a*) change leukocytes so that they become sticky, attach to the wall of a capillary, and migrate into the tissues and (*b*) cause adjacent cells to proliferate. In neither case has the chemical agent or agents responsible been identified.

This brief discussion is inserted essentially to justify what has been said about the triggerlike action of antigen on an immunologically competent cell. The effect is regarded as equivalent to a nicely adjusted degree of minor damage; although no one has a very clear idea how the liberation of these reactive agents is beneficial to the body, we can have no real doubt that they do have an important function.

There is one further topic on the cellular side of immunity that should be introduced at this stage, though it will have to be elaborated when we come to discuss the nature of antibody production in the next chapter. We have already mentioned how tuberculin sensitivity can be transferred to a nontuberculous animal by the inoculation of cells from spleen or lymph nodes. Serum is quite ineffective. The same holds when we are concerned not with the simple transfer of antibody from one animal to another but with transfer of the capacity to make antibody.

If we have a stock of inbred mice so uniform genetically that they will accept grafts of skin or other organs from one another, we are in a much better position to carry out such experiments than if we use randomly bred animals. If we transfer serum from an immunized animal to a normal one, the amount detectable in the blood (its antibody titer) falls rapidly, the antibody being distributed more or less equally between blood and tissues. Once this redistribution is completed the titer falls more slowly, its value diminishing to half each 4 to 5 days until it becomes undetectable. If then the mouse is given a single dose of antigen there is only the low-level response of any normal mouse. If, on the other hand, spleen cells from an immunized animal are transferred, there is a variable production of antibody, usually appearing 4 to 7 days after transfer of the cells and falling more slowly. If the animals are tested with an injection of antigen 3 to 6 months later, when their antibody titer is nil or very low, they will respond in secondary fashion, that is, with a more rapid and a larger response than is ever obtained from normal mice. This experiment has the important implication that all the "information" needed to allow antibody production can be transferred from the spleen of an immune animal. Clearly neither the nervous system nor the blood vessels have anything to do with storing the information that allows a secondary response months or years later.

5. The Cellular Background

The process of embryonic development by which a fertilized egg becomes a man, a mouse, or a chicken can be described with considerable accuracy and detail at the level of gross and microscopic anatomy. Some of the biochemical changes taking place during some phases of this differentiation into tissues and organs have been put on record. But of the process by which the information stored in the chromosomes of the initiating cell is expressed progressively in form and function, we know almost nothing.

Our ignorance of this fundamental process of differentiation is a major obstacle to progress. Every problem in medicine — not least the nature of immunity — will be easier to tackle with each improvement in our understanding of differentiation.

In the history of science, help toward the understanding of an apparently insoluble central problem has sometimes been gained from some success in a peripheral or applied field. If immunology cannot draw much from what is known of the general process of differentiation and development in the embryo, it is still possible that an immunological approach, using its own concepts, might provide a clue to what happens in the wider field. In this chapter we are concerned more closely with the cells responsible for immune reactions than we have previously been. These cells, like every other cell in the body, have a developmental history: they are differentiated and to some extent specialized descendants of the fertilized ovum. One of the fascinations of speculative immunology is the hope that the special quality of immunological competence may allow us to understand how this arose in development and perhaps how it is related to more general processes of differentiation.

Early in the process of embryonic development there appear between the epithelial layers unspecialized ameboid cells which have no part in the construction of the organs. These are mesenchymal cells, from which most histologists believe all types of mobile cells that are present in the grown animal have been derived. These include the red cells of the blood and the various types of circulating leukocyte. As well as the cells actually circulating in the blood, similar cells are concentrated at three major sites, either because they are sites of proliferation in which new individual cells are produced, or because a concentration there is needed for the proper functioning of the body. These are the thymus, where in the child most lymphocytes seem to be produced; the bone marrow, which is responsible for the production of red cells and the granular leukocytes of the blood; and the spleen and the lymph nodes, scattered at strategic points through the body. In addition, there are many regions, particularly along the alimentary canal and including especially the tonsils and the appendix, where these mesenchymal cells are accumulated presumably to carry out some significant function. Finally, we have in total a vast population of cells, mostly lymphocytes, in the interstices of all tissues of the body.

There is an important minority opinion becoming heard that the striking association of lymphocytes with what are originally derivatives of endodermal epithelium, such as thymus, tonsil, and, in birds, the bursa of Fabricius, may indicate that the lymphocytes or some of them are not mesenchymal derivatives but are descended from cells of endodermal origin. This view is an attractive one, but the great majority of immunologists would undoubtedly prefer to accept a "unitarian" hypothesis, that the lymphocyte and all the other mobile cells are of mesenchymal origin.

Throughout the life of the animal, from the period when the main pattern of the body is first laid down, there are present primitive-looking undifferentiated cells, which are called by many names, stem cell or blast being those in widest colloquial use in the laboratories. Such cells have a large, loosely textured nucleus and a moderate amount of cytoplasm in which there is often evidence of active protein synthesis.

There is general agreement that these are the cells from which stem all the variety of specialized mesenchymal cells. When one looks at smears or sections taken from the proper place at the proper time, all gradations of appearance between the common stem cell and the typical end products, such as the granular leukocyte, the small lymphocyte, and the red cell, can be found. Despite the difficulty of understanding how a single cell can, under some unknown differentiating stimulus, give rise to lines ending in any one of these very different cells, few histologists have any doubts that this is what does happen.

In dealing with immunology, we can neglect the red cell completely except as something acted on by immune processes, and except in very specialized contexts we can also pass by the different sorts of granular leukocytes which play the main role in dealing with acute bacterial infection. There are three sorts of cell with which we are primarily concerned: the lymphocyte, the plasma cell, and the monocyte. It is accepted that these are all ultimately derived by descent from the stem cell and that intermediate forms — often designated by the suffix — *blast* — such as lymphoblasts or plasmablasts, can be found in appropriate situations.

The three types and their precursors may be briefly described, mainly from the functional standpoint.

(1) The small lymphocyte is one of the most ubiquitous cells in the body. It accounts for 30 to 40 percent of the white cells in the blood and is the commonest cell in thymus, lymph nodes, and spleen. Enormous numbers are present in the lining membranes of throat and bowel and appreciable numbers will be found wandering through almost every tissue in the body. The small lymphocyte has a densely staining nucleus of normal size but only a thin rim of cytoplasm, which, apart from a few small granules (mitochondria), contains no vestige of functional machinery that can be seen in sections made for electron microscopy. In current textbooks it is stated that the function of the lymphocyte is unknown but most present-day workers in immunology feel that in some way it must play a major part in immune processes. In the clonal-selection theory of immunity, to be discussed in Chapter 7, it plays a key role as the carrier of immunological "information" and as the source from which, under appropriate circumstances, new stem cells derive.

(2) The plasma cell is the main, perhaps the only, producer of antibody and gamma globulin. In sections conventionally stained, it has a nucleus whose chromatin tends to be accumulated in lumps at the periphery, giving a so-called cartwheel appearance. The cytoplasm is extensive and stains darkly with

basic dyes. In the combination of methyl green and pyronin (Unna-Pappenheim stain) which is much used in this field of work, the cytoplasm of both plasma cells and their immature precursors stains deeply red, indicating the presence of large amounts of ribonucleic acid (RNA), which is the chief intermediary in the process of protein synthesis. Heavy staining with pyronin is therefore taken as an indication that globulin or some other protein is being actively produced in the cell. In sections photographed in the electron microscope, the cytoplasm is crowded with the characteristic protein synthetic structure, the ergastoplasm or endoplasmic reticulum, often vesiculated and sometimes even showing crystalline gamma globulin within the vesicles. Mitochondria are also numerous and in a perinuclear area the ergastoplasm is displaced by the Golgi body, whose presence is another indication of high metabolic activity. It is clearly a highly active cell, elaborately tooled to produce globulin molecules and contrasting strikingly with the tenuity and emptiness of the lymphocyte's cytoplasm.

(3) The monocyte in the blood is the equivalent of the macrophage in the spleen and other tissues. It has a large nucleus, often kidney shaped, and plentiful cytoplasm of a typical finely granular texture. These cells can appear in a wide range of size and form, but their common functional characteristic is their ability to take in a variety of particulate material, from bacteria to large-molecule dyes, by phagocytosis. From the distribution of such cells we could predict that they played an important part in bodily defense against bacteria, and 60 or 70 years of experimental study has established their importance in this respect.

In their typical form each of these cells is unmistakable, but, whenever one looks at a smear or a section from spleen, bone marrow, lymph node, or some area of not particularly acute inflammation, one will always find cells difficult or impossible to classify. It is natural, therefore, to think that sometimes one of these types can change into another, and a great deal of discussion has centered on the limitations of change as between the various histological types of mesenchymal cells. Most histologists would probably agree that if for any reason one of their colleagues would be happy to find that cell type x can change into cell type y he will almost certainly be able to find convincing-looking intermediates somewhere.

A simple working approach can be developed, which has not been proved true but which has equally not been disallowed by past studies. The red cell and the granular leukocytes are specialized cells which when they have once started on their path cannot turn back. They are end cells which can have no descendants. The three types with which we are specially concerned, however, can be regarded as functional modifications within a rather generalized type of mesenchymal cell, none of which are completely precluded from further development and proliferation. There is probably only a very small chance that a small lymphocyte will ever take on a form which will allow it to have descendants, but there are 10^{13} lymphocytes in the human body and if only 1/10,000 of them give rise to new clones of cells they could play a vital part in immunity. The mature plasma cell may be an end cell which persists inert for long periods, but virtually nothing seems to be known about what happens to the plasma cells, which appear in vast numbers during an active secondary immune response. The macrophage has no set life story and most histologists would allot it extensive possibilities of new development.

The view we shall adopt, then, is that the lymphocyte is probably a carrier of genetic information, the plasma cell a producer of antibody, and the macrophage a general scavenger of unwanted material, but that all spring from the same stem cells and on appropriate stimulation can, on occasion, be converted into or give rise to stem cells from which a descendant clone can derive.

The word "clone" is used in botany for a population of plants descended from a single individual by vegetative (nonsexual) propagation (Fig. 3). It is equally applicable to any

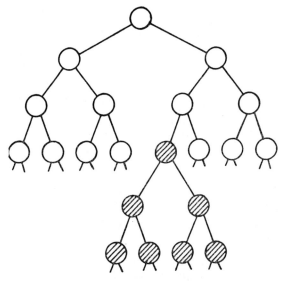

Fig. 3. To illustrate the concept of a clone as the descendants from a single cell or organism. Any mutation or other inheritable change is taken as initiating a new clone.

organism or cell that multiplies without at any stage interchanging genetic material with another unit. The word is used extensively in discussions of the cells concerned in immunity primarily because, as has already been mentioned, cells appear to be able to transmit something we can call immunological memory to their descendants. It is now generally accepted that cells which for one reason or another have become competent to react with a certain antigen can produce descendants which will retain that capacity to "recognize" this antigen. All cells which by this type of relation have a common immunological character comprise a clone.

Protein synthesis

When a well-defined antigen, a blood protein like bovine serum albumin (BSA) or a virus like influenza, is injected on more than one occasion, so that a sharp secondary response with active antibody production is in progress, many plasma cells are always to be found in the lymph nodes that drain the area of injection. One would expect that they were producing the antibody and by a special histological method, Coons's sandwich technique, one can show that they *are* making the antibody and, further, that if the body is engaged in making two sorts of antibody each plasma cell is making one or the other, not both. Coons's technique is an ingenious one, depending on the fact that one can attach a fluorescent dye to an antibody molecule so that, wherever the antibody aggregates, a corresponding area of fluorescence will be visible in a properly illuminated section. If we have fluorescent antibody available as well as antigen and we are examining plasma cells which may be producing antibody, we can establish this by first treating a section of the lymph node with the antigen. If antibody is being made by the cell, there will be enough on its cut surface to bind the antigen to it. Excess antigen is now washed away and the section is treated with fluorescent antibody. This in its turn unites with free groupings on the bound antigen molecules, completing the sandwich. Any plasma cell that glows with the proper color under the microscope can therefore be identified with certainty as being engaged in production of antibody similar to that combined with the fluorescent dye.

Antibody, then, is a protein synthesized by the plasma cell in much the same way that trypsinogen is made in a cell of the pancreas. Both types of cell seen in section under the electron microscope contain an elaborate structure of double sheets and vesicles, the ergastoplasm, within which mass synthesis can take place. There is also no reason to doubt that the actual process of synthesis is similar to that by which all the countless proteins, especially enzymes needed in the cell, are synthesized.

Enzymes have much in common with antibodies, and all theories of antibody production have of necessity had to pay much attention to the more accessible field of study provided by bacterial enzymes. Both enzymes and antibodies can be looked at as large protein molecules, small areas of which are specially constructed to make a close-fitting union with another rather small chemical configuration. An enzyme undergoes union with its substrate as a preliminary to its catalytic action. An antibody unites to the corresponding antigen without inducing any direct chemical change.

Before going further it is advisable to add a little more to what has already been said about the physical nature of antigens and antibodies. The most important point is that the active group of an antibody, what we shall call its specific pattern, is quite small, covering an area (estimated to be about 100 to 200 square angstroms) within which a large but by no means unlimited variety of configurations could be formed. There are probably two such special areas on each antibody molecule, and there is some evidence that a proportion of molecules may have one or three areas. In the same way the antigenic determinants with which the specific patterns of the antibody combine are also molecular configurations usually represented several times over the surface of any large antigenic molecule. It is by no means clear what portion of any given protein or other organic macromolecule is potentially antigenic. It is a useful and possibly correct assumption that any macromolecule has a complex surface mosaic of potential antigenic determinants. Whether or not any one of them will actually function will depend (*a*) on its absence from the components of the body of the animal being considered as antibody producer, and (*b*) on its macromolecular or other carrier having the qualities necessary for antigenicity.

It is tacitly accepted that the structure of all the protein molecules which make up the tissues and fluids of the body is determined in the last analysis by the genetic information carried in the fertilized ovum and transferred by mitosis to all descendant cells. At the present time the central aim of biochemistry is to understand the connections between the genetic information and the chemical constitution of the specific protein which eventually appears.

This is not the place to attempt a summary of the rapidly developing picture of protein synthesis. All that need be said is that interpretations in 1961 placed the primary genetic information in the desoxyribonucleic acid (DNA) and ascribed the code in which it was expressed to the distribution of purine-pyrimidine bases in the linear model of DNA due to Watson and Crick. This, by a process involving RNA as an intermediary, provided a means by which amino acids were united in a determinate sequence into a polypeptide chain. The differences between proteins were presumed to depend wholly on the sequence of amino acids and the length of the chain. No protein exists in the form of a simple linear polypeptide, but the simplest form of present theory considers that the initial sequence will determine a unique way in which the protein molecule will fold into a globular, spiral, or other form.

All biochemists are convinced of the overriding importance of amino acid sequence in determining the nature of a protein, but an influential group will not accept that it uniquely determines the secondary folding of the molecule. They believe that there are many possibilities of secondary modification, such as the control of folding by a secondary template of genetic origin or the combination of a polypeptide chain with other units, whether of peptide or other structure, determined by separate genetic factors.

Some such formulation is almost obligatory in relation to antibody. In the rabbit and perhaps in other animals, all gamma globulin has a common component in the form of an easily crystallized protein comprising about 40 percent of the globulin molecule, which can be split off by light treatment with the enzyme papain. Two other fractions, a little smaller in size, carry the specific pattern of the antibody. No decision has been reached as to whether the specific pattern is laid down as a special sequence of amino acids during the primary formation of the polypeptide chain or whether it results from a secondary modification of genetic or other origin. It is at this level that controversy between the holders of different theories of antibody formation arises.

Population dynamics

The healthy body is a self-regulating system of extreme complexity. When dealing with the mesenchymal cells we have one of the simpler problems of control, since these are mobile cells often packed temporarily into solid tissues but not playing an active part in the architecture of the body. The most conspicuous of the cells which we have taken as our special concern is the lymphocyte. In a healthy individual around 30 percent of the white blood cells are lymphocytes, 3000 per cubic millimeter and a total of 20,000,000,000 (2×10^{10}), in the whole of the blood. In lymph nodes, spleen, and the tissues generally there are 300–500 times as many as this, or

10^{13}. These numbers remain approximately constant, yet there is good evidence that about 5×10^{11} new lymphocytes are produced each day; hence there must necessarily be about the same number lost or destroyed. In the rat and probably other mammals, the most important source of new lymphocytes is the thymus gland. In the young, where the need is apparently highest, the thymus is larger and more active than in older animals. The thymus contains a hormone which increases the number of lymphocytes in the blood when administered to baby mice and which may well be one of the instruments of control to maintain the standard population levels of lymphocytes in the body. Lymph nodes, spleen, tonsils, appendix, and the lymphoid accumulations of the intestine are also important sources of new lymphocytes. To anticipate later stages of the discussion a little, it seems possible that the thymus is the center of production of "virgin" lymphocytes whose ancestors have not had immunological experience, while the other centers produce most of the lymphocytes that carry immunological memories from their precursors.

In the centers of lymphocyte production one finds stem cells and a sequence of large, medium, and small lymphocytes which represent successive changes of appearance with multiplication. Once the typical small lymphocyte appears, it ceases to multiply and either passes to the blood or is retained in crowded masses around the centers of production.

The method of autoradiography has provided a new and powerful tool for tracing the sequence and movement of cells. The most commonly used technique depends on the fact that thymidine is an essential component of DNA and wherever synthesis of DNA is occurring thymidine present in the environment will be taken up into the nucleus. If radioactive thymidine carrying the isotope tritium (H^3) is provided, it will be incorporated into all cells actively synthesizing DNA.

The standard technique is to inject tritiated thymidine into a series of animals in a single intravenous dose. At appropriate periods films or sections are prepared from the animals and mounted in the dark against a sensitive photographic film. After a few weeks in the dark each cell which has taken up the labeled thymidine produces an effect on the photographic emulsion which, when the film is developed, appears as dark granules of silver over the nucleus. In this way it is possible to follow the descendants of cells which took up the radioisotope by recognizing their radioactivity and assessing to what degree it has been reduced by growth and multiplication. The results have indicated the high reproductive activity of the stem cells and have confirmed the recognized sequence of forms to the fully developed granulocyte and small lymphocyte, as well as giving a time scale to the sequence. It takes about six divisions and 3 to 4 days for a small lymphocyte to be derived from a stem cell.

By a variety of methods it has been shown that the average life of a given lymphocyte in the circulation is only a matter of hours. Individual cells are constantly passing out of the circulation into the tissues, whence many of them are collected into lymph nodes and eventually to the main lymphatic vessels which deliver a mixture of new and old lymphocytes into the blood. Many lymphocytes leak out into the lining membranes of intestine and respiratory tract and are lost in the body. Many others just seem to disappear. Any form of stress, or, what perhaps amounts to the same thing, administration of large doses of cortisone and similar corticosteroid hormones, will sharply reduce the number of lymphocytes in blood and in the lymphoid tissues. Apparently the cells are very easily damaged and then digest themselves and disintegrate. Their components are then available again for use in the body, perhaps particularly in the tissue where disintegration occurs. Some histologists think it likely that these fragments of lymphocytic nuclei may be valuable "building material" for the construction of new cells in the germinal centers of the lymph nodes.

Finally, both histological and experimental evidence suggests that some lymphocytes, no doubt those in the less active areas of lymph nodes and elsewhere, may retain their identity for a year or more.

This covers, superficially at least, the life history of the lymphocyte as it is known at present. The chief points to be recognized are (*a*) the constant turnover of lymphocytes, (*b*) the variability in their individual lifetimes, which may range from a few hours to 300 or 400 days, and (*c*) the existence of some degree of recirculation.

There are, however, some crucially important gaps in our knowledge. We have only the most limited information about how the level of lymphocytes in the blood is maintained or why lymph nodes and spleen stay approximately constant in size. There is clear evidence that part of the control is hormonal in character, thymus extracts accelerating their production and the corticosteroids from the adrenal favoring their destruction. Nothing is known about the regulatory mechanism or the nature of the "feedback" which must activate it. The second great gap is our ignorance in regard to potentialities of interconversion between different types of mesenchymal cells. An interpretation favored by some authorities is that medium and small lymphocytes when they reach a favorable situation in the body, notably the bone marrow, can be converted to an undifferentiated stem cell which can give rise to a whole clone of descendant lymphocytes (and perhaps other types of cell). Others hold that once a small lymphocyte is in existence it has no further potentiality of development — it is a typical end cell. Unfortunately from the point of view of clarifying the situation experimentally, not more than 1 in 100 or 1 in 1000 cells would need to undergo de-differentiation to the stem-cell form to produce the descendants needed to maintain the lymphocyte population. It will always be difficult and perhaps impossible to demonstrate a rare process of this sort by histological methods. Indirect evidence will have to provide most of the support for our belief in the reality of the process.

Plasma cells, the characteristic producers of antibody, can be found in small numbers in all normal animals past the first week or two of life. Wherever antibody is being actively produced they are found in large numbers in the relevant lymphoid organs. Clear sequences can be followed from stem cell to mature plasma cell, more or less parallel to the sequence of large, medium, and small lymphocytes. It has also been claimed that large and medium lymphocytes and monocytes can be converted directly to forms in the plasma-cell series. In animals that have been heavily immunized it is common to find numerous mature plasma cells which contain bodies that are probably highly concentrated and sometimes crystallized antibody globulin. These seem to be quiescent terminal cells. Nothing is known of the normal fate of plasma cells. After the height of a secondary antibody response they diminish in number, but whether this is by destruction and absorption or by conversion to another type is unknown. Plasma cells are only very rarely found in the blood.

Macrophages — often called histiocytes or cells of the reticuloendothelial system when in the tissues, and monocytes in the blood — are the scavengers of the body. At one stage in the development of immunology it was regarded as almost self-evident that these were the cells responsible for immunity. If dead bacteria are injected into the circulation or into the tissues, most of them will be taken up by macrophages, just as any finely divided mineral or other insoluble particles will be. It seemed highly likely, therefore, that to take in and digest foreign microorganisms and toxins was the first step toward the production of antibody. At the present time, however, most immunologists tend to neglect the macrophage and deny that it has any direct role in antibody production. They do not, of course, deny its importance as one of the agents of immunity, but regard its phagocytic activity as a physiological rather than an immunological function. There are one or two observations which do suggest that some macrophages

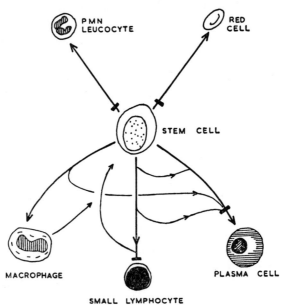

Fig. 4. A schematic diagram of the origin of the cells concerned with immunity. The heavy lines mark the normal course of development, lighter ones the direction of possible interconversions of one type into another. The bars indicate points beyond which conversion to another type is believed to be impossible. PMN leucocyte: polymorphonuclear leukocyte of the blood.

have a special capacity to take up one particular kind of particle, but they are not clear enough to serve as a basis for any general statement.

It would be hopeless to attempt to discuss the varied opinions that have been expressed on the origin and potentialities of the macrophages. Instead we can adopt a simplified picture, which is admittedly not rigorously established and which can well be regarded as being chosen to fit into a particular theory of immunity rather than on its intrinsic merits. Nevertheless there is no indication from observation or experiment that it is either untenable or unlikely. On this view the mesenchymal cells represent a differentiated population of cells which has become specialized to respond to appropriate stimuli within the internal environment of the body by switching to one or other type of development and eventual function. The capacity to respond varies with the physiological state of the cell, and once a cell line has moved too far along a particular path it may be incapable of being diverted. The appearances which we call lymphocyte, plasma cell, or monocyte are on this view just a morphological expression of the particular function that a mesenchymal cell has been stimulated to perform. Figure 4 is an attempt to express the relations of these cell types in diagrammatic form.

6. Self-recognition

On several occasions already it has been noted that no ordinary component of the body will provoke an immunological response. Antibody production or any other type of immunological reaction is against foreign material — against something that is not self.

The classical example is drawn from human experience with skin grafting. It is known to all surgeons that skin can readily be grafted from one site to another on the same individual. Skin grafting of this type is in everyday use for the repair of burnt areas of skin and many other types of damage by injury or disease. If an attempt is made to use skin from another individual, there will usually be a period of a week or thereabouts during which the graft will become attached and, for a day or two, appear pink and healthy. Then, however, the graft becomes inflamed, darkens, and begins to separate, the blood connection fails, and the graft is rejected as a distorted scab. The body is clearly rejecting tissue that in some way it can recognize as foreign to itself.

The "Rh-baby" story that was described in Chapter 3 is clearly of similar character, but perhaps it is easier to see the implications of blood-group differences in a different fashion. Suppose we have three men available for an experiment, two of them, A and B, Rh-negative and the third, C, Rh-positive; to eliminate other complications we shall assume that all are of the same ABO blood group. None of them at the beginning of the experiment have any antibody against the red blood cells of any of the others and, of course, none against their own. Subject A (Rh-negative) is injected with 1 ml of blood B (also Rh-negative) and the injection is repeated a month later. Tests of his serum show no action on blood cells A, B, or C. After that experiment is completed, A receives an injection of C's blood (Rh-positive). Nothing happens after the first injection but after the second he feels a little off color and shivery for an hour or two. A fortnight later his blood serum will clump a suspension of C's red cells even when it is diluted over 100 times but has no action on his own or B's cells. To complete the experiment we must test what happens when C is inoculated with blood from another Rh-positive subject, D, and when Rh-negative blood is injected into an Rh-positive individual. All the results would be negative, but if we persevered with injecting Rh-negative blood into Rh-positive people we might eventually obtain a serum which was without action on C and D (Rh-positive) but did agglutinate A and B (Rh-negative).

In outline this is the way in which all the blood groups except ABO have been sorted out except for the fact that the "injection" of foreign blood was usually by way of pregnancy or therapeutic transfusion. It is clear that Rh-positive blood cells carry an antigenic component which in persons without that component can provoke an antibody but cannot do so in anyone who possesses it. Rh-negative individuals who lack this factor have in its place another, which, however, is far less antigenic than its Rh-positive equivalent.

From this series of experiments we can make a provisional generalization which, in fact, seems to be valid for all but a few very rare situations. An individual human or animal will not produce antibody or show any other immunological reaction against antigenic patterns present in its cells or body fluids, provided these are not functionally insulated from the general turnover of cells in the body. The important potential exceptions include some components of the brain and spinal cord, the eye, the testis, thyroid and adrenal glands, and possibly some other endocrine glands. Foreign patterns not represented in the accessible tissues may but do not necessarily provoke antibody. One of the main problems we shall have to discuss is why some antigens like the Rh-positive factor D are good antigens, easily stimulating antibody production, while others produce antibody only with the greatest difficulty.

The other important aspect which has become clear largely as a result of studies on blood groups is the regularity of their inheritance. The antigens appear to correspond in a one-to-one fashion to the genes, so that studies on the inheritance of the blood groups have become a favorite occupation for geneticists.

As is the rule in genetic studies, most of the blood groups when they were first discovered seemed to have rather simple genetic relationships, but as experience widened progressive complications emerged. Here it would be merely academic pedantry to attempt a full account, but it is worth indicating the simple rules of the ABO and the Rh groups as they were before the rarer exceptions complicated, but did not seriously modify, the significance of the early formulation.

In the ABO group we have four blood groups which can be determined in the laboratory: O, A, B, and AB. These are the phenotypes. The corresponding genetic structures are based on the assumption that there are three possible alleles (alternative forms) A, B, and O for a certain gene on one chromosome and that either A or B is dominant to O. Table 3 shows that AB and O can have only one genotype but that persons reported as A or B can have either two similar genes or one with the gene *O* on the corresponding second chromosome.

Table 3. *Simplified table of the common ABO and Rh blood groups.*

Blood group (phenotype)	Genotypes	Approximate frequency in England (percent)
AB	A/B	3
A	A/A A/O	42
B	B/B B/O	8.5
O	O/O	46.5
Rh+	CDe/CDe	16.6 ⎫
	CDe/cDE	11.5 ⎪
	CDe/cde	31 ⎬ 84.9
	CDE/cDE	2 ⎪
	cDE/cde	11 ⎭
Rh−	cde/cde	15.1

The Rh situation is more complex, with three adjacent points on a chromosome, each of which can be occupied by one or more alleles. Each gene represents one antigenic pattern on a red cell and all genes on both chromosomes of the individual are represented in the red-cell structure. There are only three really common combinations: CDe, cde, cDE. Since it is the presence or absence of D which determines Rh-positive and Rh-negative reactions, all Rh-negative people are of the genotype cde/cde. In the table only the six common combinations are shown; there are also probably more than 100 rare ones.

This somewhat detailed discussion of blood-group inheritance is intended to provide a justification for the broader generalization that all the complex macromolecules of the body carry antigenic patterns whose configuration is wholly determined by the information carried in the genetic make-up of the organism. It is an intimidating thought that there is more information on organic chemical synthesis packed into the head of a spermatozoon than in all the 200 volumes of *The Journal of Biological Chemistry.*

Any approach, however superficial, to the understanding of immunology must be based on what is known of the way in which information in the genetic mechanism is translated into the production of molecules of protein, polysaccharide, and so forth, each carrying a predetermined chemical pattern. Since antibodies are proteins, it is the synthesis of protein which will chiefly concern us. There is an even more important reason for giving proteins preeminence. The construction of all types of organic molecule in the body, including protein itself, is the work of specific enzymes, and all enzymes consist either wholly or predominantly of protein. For technical reasons it is often simpler to detect and measure small amounts of an enzyme than of any other type of protein, and much of the basic research on protein synthesis has been concerned with the synthesis of enzymes.

As in so many other situations, it is practicable to present only a simplified picture, which must be false in detail and may even eventually be proved wrong in principle. I believe that in 1960 most biochemists would accept the picture to be given as acceptable for its particular purpose.

The information in the genes and chromosomes of the genetic machinery is carried in a kind of code based on the fact that the long molecules of nucleic acid are built up of sequences of four different sorts of units. A, G, T, C are the initials of the names of these units but perhaps it is simpler to replace them by 1, 2, 3, 4. A nucleic acid filament is a double spiral structure in which the two threads have a special relation to each other, but for the present we can concentrate on one only of these threads. It might have the sequence 1 1 2 1 4 4 3 4 1 1 4 1 2 3 2 1 3 3 1 4 4. Obviously, with a little ingenuity, a code could be devised by which such a sequence could be used to convey a message in cryptic form. In fact what is required is that such a coded sequence should be capable of telling in what order an entirely different sort of linear sequence should be constructed. Here instead of 4 sorts of units we have 20 sorts of units that will need to be arranged to give as it were a correct translation of the first message. Proteins are built up of amino acids, of which there are 20 types commonly present in proteins with 8 more which may be found in special circumstances. Present opinion is that the character of a protein is almost wholly determined by the sequence and number of amino acids that are built into the

Table 4. *One possible code for protein synthesis.*

A 112		I 141	O 241	T 341
B 212		L 142	P 242	U 342
		M 143	R 243	V 343
C 131	F 231	N 144	S 244	W 344
D 132	G 232			
E 133	H 233			

primary linear macromolecules, usually called the polypeptide chain. In some way, then, the four-symbol code of the nucleic acid must be capable of ordering the sequence of amino acids in the protein whose structure it controls.

It can be shown that if one takes the four symbols in triplets it is possible to choose 20 triplets which, when arranged in sequences, will always give an unambiguous interpretation. There are many ways of getting 20 triplets but in each there are only 20 which will fill the requirements. One set is shown in Table 4. We can use 20 of the letters of the alphabet to correspond one with each triplet and then set out the word BLOOD as 212142241241132. Even if this were embedded in a meaningless sequence at both ends it would still be unambiguously interpretable as BLOOD.

Theoretically minded biochemists now suggest that a protein is synthesized by a process involving *first* the linkage of an amino acid A to a small length of nucleic acid including the triplet 112. The triplet then clicks into place with its corresponding triplet in the ordered sequence on the nucleic acid chain and holds the amino acid in the right position for a process of linking to those on either side by means of appropriate enzymes (see Fig. 5). This, of course, is a grossly oversimplified picture, but it is at least provisionally helpful in showing the intrinsic reasonableness of the view that information is transferred in the process of protein synthesis. There has been a deliberate omission of many aspects of much current interest. No mention has been made of the difference between DNA, the type of nucleic acid that carries the genetic codes, and the other type, RNA, which seems to be responsible for the actual synthesis of protein. Since no detail has been introduced, one can hope that the present rather naïve account may continue to be acceptable (of its genre) when much more information is available about the detailed chemistry of the process.

From our present point of view, the important implication of these experiments and ideas is that in general the detailed specification of a protein, whether antigen, enzyme, or globulin, is carried in the genetic structure of the cell or organism. In general, where the capacity of a cell or an organism to produce a recognizable protein can be shown to be inherited, then we have a prima-facie case for the pattern of that protein being determined at the genetic level. The modern concept makes it reasonable that immunological recognition

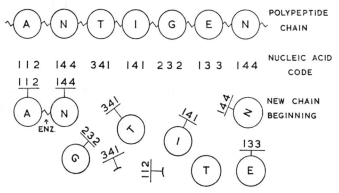

Fig. 5. A diagram to represent one interpretation of the process of protein synthesis (greatly simplified). The individual amino acids which will be built into the polypeptide chain of a protein are shown as A, N, . . . Corresponding to each type of amino acid is a "soluble RNA" which can act as a carrier to bring it to the right position in the sequence because of its pattern correspondence with the appropriate portion of the nucleic acid code. An enzyme (ENZ) then forms the peptide bond.

of self should be genetically based. It is not recognition of self as such but of genetically determined uniformity of chemical pattern. A skin graft will take on a person's own body but it will take equally well on his identical twin and an identical twin is identical simply because the twins derived from the same fertilized ovum are genetic replicas. In mice that have been closely enough inbred, we can obtain the same genetic uniformity. They are isogenic and will accept skin grafts from one another.

An indication of how close genetic resemblance must be to allow tolerance of each other's tissues can be gained from considering the results of cross-grafting skin between different sexes of closely inbred mice. Sex is a genetic character and a male and a female can never be wholly isogenic. In mice and other mammals the male can be represented by XY and the female by XX. The male Y chromosome can influence the production of some protein patterns not produced in the female but all the patterns that the female can produce can also be produced by the male. On experimental test it is found that in most inbred strains male will accept male skin and female female. Males will accept female skin because nothing foreign is being introduced but females (XX) will not so readily accept male skin (XY), which contains those foreign elements sponsored by genes in the Y chromosome.

Tolerance

We have already discussed some of Nature's experiments in which during embryonic life the blood circulation of two genetically dissimilar twins fuses and allows each to develop a tolerance of the other's cells. The same phenomenon can be studied experimentally by prenatal injection of suitable animals.

Suppose we have two stocks of mice, A (white) and B (black), both so closely inbred that they will freely accept grafts from another of the same stock but not, of course, one from the opposite group. In our first experiment we take a pregnant A mouse near term and inject each of the embryos with living cells taken from B embryos of the same age; spleen and kidney cells are normally used. If all goes well, the injected A embryos are born naturally and develop normally. At 6 or 8 weeks of age — late adolescence for a mouse — each is grafted with B skin. In most or all, the graft takes and we have the biological absurdity of a white mouse with a black patch of healthy foreign skin (Fig. 6). These we can call A^B mice. The capacity to tolerate foreign skin is strictly limited to the stock from which the prenatal injection was obtained. If we have a third stock C of brown inbred mice, skin from

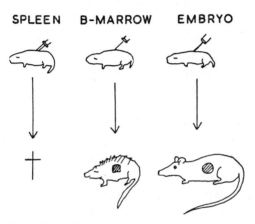

Fɪɢ. 6. The effect of injecting cells from mice of one strain B (black) into newborn mice of strain A (white). If embryonic cells are used, the mouse becomes tolerant and accepts a subsequent graft of black skin. The embryonic B cells implanted in A also persist and acquire tolerance to those antigens of the host which are foreign to them. If adult cells are used, the host learns to tolerate them but mature B cells react against the host, giving either runt disease or death.

one of these will be just as readily rejected by the A^B mouse as by a normal A mouse. The tolerance of an A^B mouse for a B skin graft lasts at least 4 months and may last for the whole life of the mouse — about 2 years.

There are various ways in which this experiment can be done, and with certain technical refinements it is possible to induce tolerance by an injection made on the first day of life but not later. There are two experiments that are of special interest for any theoretical interpretation of this phenomenon of immunological tolerance.

The first is very simple: we take a group of A^B mice carrying their black patches of skin and to half of them we graft cells from the spleen or lymph nodes of a normal A mouse. The other A^B mice remain as untreated "controls." In 2 or 3 weeks the black patches on the A^B mice that received the lymphoid cells begin to look unhealthy. The hair stops growing and eventually the foreign skin scabs off. Meanwhile the control animals continue to tolerate their grafts. This experiment is important (a) because it underlines the fact that the tolerance must be induced in the first day of life or before birth, but clearly cannot be transferred to adult lymphoid cells from another animal; (b) it indicates that the black graft is still foreign and has not been, as it were, adopted and changed to A-type cells, but can still stimulate A cells to destroy it; and (c) it suggests that tolerance is due not to some additional quality but to the loss of some normal quality that can be replaced by a nontolerant group of cells.

The second type of experiment is precisely similar to the prototype experiment for inducing tolerance but instead of injecting a litter of newborn mice with embryonic cells we use an emulsion of cells from adult spleens of B mice. One or two of the litter are left uninjected as controls. After 2 or 3 weeks it becomes evident that the injected mice are not as healthy as the uninjected. They are smaller, their hair does not lie smoothly, and they have a sticky diarrhea. Most of them die before they are 2 months old. In the laboratories this condition is known colloquially as "runt disease." If the survivors are test grafted with B skin, the graft will survive. The animals are tolerant to the foreign cells, but the adult foreign cells will not tolerate their host. This seems to be the reason for runt disease. It is, of course, only logical that when cells from two individuals are compelled to live together each sort must become tolerant of the other. If this is simplest when the animal is very young, then obviously we are likely to get our best results by bringing both sorts of cell together in the late embryonic period, just as takes place in natural chimeras.

All the experiments that have been described have made use of cells — living cells of another individual — to induce tolerance. For further analysis of the process we need to use a pure protein and for convenience in the type of work required, a larger animal, the rabbit. Very pure samples of blood serum albumin, either human or bovine, are now available commercially and bovine serum albumin, BSA, is the protein most commonly used in immunological experiments.

No animal can produce antibody till it is at least 14 days old but after that the full capacity builds up rapidly. At 3 months a normal rabbit shows a well-defined response to an injection of BSA in the standard dose — 100 mg per kilogram of body weight. The amount of antigen in the blood falls at a steady rate for about a week and then falls much more steeply (Fig. 7). Just at this stage antibody begins to appear and there are easily detectable amounts within 3 weeks. If another injection of BSA is given subsequently, the full secondary response follows. The amount in the circulation falls rapidly from the start and an active production of new antibody commences within 5 days.

A rabbit given the standard dose of BSA very soon after birth, however, behaves quite differently. An injection at 3 months is followed by a smooth fall of antigen in the blood, without any acceleration toward the end of the first week, and no antibody is produced. Even more striking is the fact that a similar injection after another 3 months gives a reaction exactly similar to the first. Not only is there no secondary response, there is not even a primary one. Tolerance, in the sense of failure to give an immunological response, seems to be complete and long lasting. Smith and Bridges, who were responsible for this work found, however, that if the first test

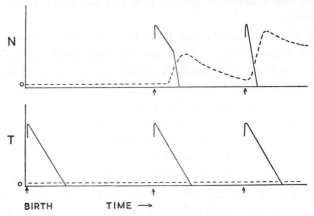

Fig. 7. To show tolerance to a soluble antigen. Two rabbits are inoculated with a protein antigen at intervals and the amounts of antigen and antibody in the blood are measured at regular intervals. The normal rabbit, N, is first inoculated at 3 months of age and shows accelerated removal of antigen and the normal antibody response. The second rabbit, T, is rendered tolerant by an inoculation of antigen on the day of birth. This produces no antibody and leaves the animal nonresponsive to the two subsequent injections of the same antigen. Solid line: concentration of antigen in the blood; broken line: concentration of antibody in the blood.

injection of BSA was given 6 months or more after the initial dose on the first day of life the rabbit responded with a normal antibody rise. It would be surprising if the amount of antigen and the time between tests did not have an important bearing on the results and detailed tests soon established this. Tolerance after 100 mg/kg persists for more than 3 months but not for 6. If a second injection is given within the period of tolerance, this is extended for another period of about the same length and the process can be continued indefinitely. If the initial dose is 10 mg/kg, tolerance lasts for a much shorter time. Smith and Bridges give good reasons for believing that tolerance is possible only so long as the antigen persists in the body.

Any protein like BSA is eventually broken down and elim- inated, irrespective of whether the animal can develop im- munity or not. A population of cells implanted in fetal life can persist indefinitely and it is a reasonable deduction that tolerance in such a case depends on the continuing liberation of foreign antigen by the implanted cells. There is one other type of agent which can theoretically be introduced into the embryo and persist into adult life. This is a virus of appro- priate low-grade activity. There is only one example that has been adequately studied, a virus disease of mice which can occasionally cause serious human infections, lymphocytic choriomeningitis (LCM). A laboratory infection indicated the probability that one of the Rockefeller Institute's mouse stocks was infected with the virus in 1935. Traub studied the natural history of the disease in this group of mice. He found that in a heavily infected population there was very little evidence of overt disease, but, if he injected blood or tissue suspensions from any mouse of the group into normal mice free of the virus, these came down with acute disease. Here clearly was a puzzling situation that called for detailed study. After 3 years' work, Traub found that the colony was almost literally saturated with virus. Virus passed from the blood and tissue fluids of pregnant mice to the embryos in the uterus. Some of the embryos died but most were born normal. They pro- duced no antibody or other type of immune response against the virus in their tissues — just as a rabbit produces no antibody against BSA if the antigen is constantly replenished. The failure to eliminate LCM virus seems clearly to be another example of immunological tolerance. This does not, however, explain the other extraordinary feature, that a mouse which cannot produce an immune response against the virus is unharmed by it although another mouse initially free from the virus will suffer a fatal infection despite its potential capacity to become immune.

There are such interesting possibilities here that it seems worthy of a little discussion even if it means we are wandering somewhat from our proper argument. LCM virus is not a good producer of immunity, but there is a standard procedure, involving inoculation first of dead virus and then of active virus, by which mice of uninfected stock may be made fully immune. There is, however, very little antibody in the blood of these immune mice. The next clue comes from experiments in which for some reason normal mice were given a damaging dose of x-rays after being inoculated with LCM virus. Unlike the unirradiated controls, these showed no symptoms. Another way of protecting mice in basically similar fashion is to give a form of vitamin poison, an analogue of folic acid, that has a generally damaging effect on cells. Again the normal mice grow sick and die, while the damaged ones go unharmed.

The full implications of this set of phenomena are probably still to be recognized, but there are hints in the same direction in regard to other diseases. Sometimes it seems that the body's capacity to react against infection can be an embarrassment to it. In the previously healthy mouse inoculated with LCM virus in the brain, "cuffs" of cells develop around the small blood vesesls, as part of the defense reaction against the virus. No such cellular reaction occurs in the irradiated or poisoned animals. It seems that the defensive response is more dangerous than the virus it is directed against.

Perhaps one could draw a political moral here — but it would be more apposite to point out how desperately complex is the maintenance required to keep the body intact and functioning through all emergencies. The whole of the control mechanisms have had to be developed not by an infinitely intelligent designer but under the pressure of evolutionary selection. The mechanism which best allows an animal to survive the major onslaughts of potentially lethal infection may not be at all appropriate for some rare invader with a different twist to its offensiveness. Evolution must always produce the best compromise for survival; it is hardly interested in niceties.

To return to the problem of tolerance: we have seen that if, at the very beginning of independent life, foreign material, whether cells from related but genetically distinct individuals of the same species, purified foreign proteins, or a rather unusual virus, is implanted and can remain present it is likely to be accepted as "self" and no immune response will be involved against it. This capacity does not wholly cease in later life. If one gives a grown rabbit very large doses of a soluble foreign protein like BSA and continues this daily, a state is soon reached in which the rabbit cannot make anti-BSA, though it can still make antibody against an unrelated protein.

A basically similar experiment is to arrange for two genetically dissimilar mice to share each other's blood supply. There is a standard surgical technique for producing these parabiotic pairs, as they are called. By appropriate incision and suture the two mice are transformed into a pair of Siamese twins that allow the two bloods to mingle freely. If mice of the same pure strain are used, the union persists and both partners remain healthy, but with mice from an ordinary mixed stock the results will vary from pair to pair. Usually the immunological difference is too great and one or both of the partners die in a few weeks. In a proportion up to 30 or 40 percent, however, both partners survive and it has been found in one set of experiments, at least, that they have become capable of accepting a skin graft one from the other. This is a form of tolerance and must be accounted for in any theory of immunity.

"Graft-versus-host" reactions

Runt disease has already been mentioned as resulting when spleen cells from an adult mouse are injected into a day-old mouse of another strain. It depends on the fact that cells from a mature animal can become immunologically active against any type of organic pattern not present in the animal that produced them. When transferred to another environment in which they find it possible to survive, they are liable to "attack" any components of the new environment which to them are foreign.

There are, as is perhaps to be expected, considerable differences in the readiness with which runt disease is produced between two strains of mice. For our purposes we can forget about the complications of all actual experiments and speak only of two pure lines of mouse A and B which have a well-marked difference in their tissue antigens. Technically, they carry different gene alleles at the histocompatibility locus $H2$. With two strains we have three sorts of mouse to consider, A, B, and the hybrid F_1 from a cross between A and B which we can call AB. It is illuminating to summarize what we find about tissue interchange in these animals (Table 5).

The first-generation hybrid has both histocompatibility genes; since we are dealing with pure lines their genetic composition in regard to the relevant genes will be

Strain	A	B	AB
Genes	*AA*	*BB*	*AB*

and the corresponding tissue antigens will also be present.

Table 5. *Tissue reactions between two strains of mice, A and B.*

Donor	Mode of transfer	Recipient *		
		A	B	AB
A adult	Skin	Ac	R	Ac
B adult	graft to	R	Ac	Ac
AB adult	adult	R	R	Ac
A adult	Spleen	O	RD	RD
B adult	to	RD	O	RD
AB adult	newborn	O	O	O
A embryo	Spleen or	O	T	O
B embryo	kidney to	T	O	O
AB embryo	newborn	T	T	O

* Ac, graft accepted; R, graft rejected; RD, runt disease; T, tolerance; O, no demonstrable effect.

The hybrid therefore can regard both A and B antigens as self and will accept a skin graft from either parent. Incidentally, we must be careful not to draw from this the conclusion that a child can accept skin from either of his parents. All human beings are heterozygous and, as there are probably many genes involved, it would be extremely unlikely that the child would possess all the antigens of both father and mother.

On the other hand, the pure line cells A or B accepted and tolerated by the hybrid AB are, if they are of the lymphoid type, in an environment which contains a foreign component. They will therefore make mischief and produce runt disease. It should be pointed out that to produce runt disease lymphoid cells from the donor must be tolerated for an adequate length of time. If one puts adult spleen cells from A into adult mouse B or vice versa, the injected cells fail to survive and nothing obvious happens. For A cells to survive in a foreign host, that host must be either (a) less than 24 hours old, (b) irradiated sufficiently to destroy its own lymphoid tissue, or (c) a hybrid F_1 with A as one parent.

Passing from mice to chickens, we come across another interesting experimental situation. Experimentalists have known for many years that curious things happened when adult-fowl blood or cell emulsions were injected into chick embryos, but the processes have only recently been clarified. There are many ways of doing these experiments, but perhaps the simplest is to take some fowl blood into heparin solution, which prevents its coagulation, and put 0.1 ml on the chorioallantoic membrane. This is the outermost membrane of the embryo, lying immediately inside the shell and serving as a lung to bring oxygen from the air into the blood. The membrane is dropped away from the shell in the process of inoculation and the blood with its contained leukocytes is spread over about 2 in.^{2} If the membrane is examined after 4 days' further incubation, it will show something between 20 and 100 white spots, averaging about 1 mm in diameter. In another 2 or 3 days the spots will enlarge to form round white nodules from which a hard shotty center can be shelled out. At the same time the embryo's spleen will be found to be enlarged and lumpy. If the chicks are allowed to hatch, they are unhealthy from the start and die in a few days with anemia and general weakness.

This reaction, usually called the Simonsen phenomenon, has been the center of my own experimental interest for the past 2 years and I am probably overeager to draw general conclusions from the results. (Parenthetically, I have for a long time given ambitious young research workers only two pieces of general advice: "Do as large a proportion as possible of your experiments with your own hands. Always regard the topic you are working on as important both in itself

and in regard to each of the wider fields on which it bears.")
Making due allowance for such personal enthusiasm, there
are still several features of special interest in the graft-versus-
host reaction on the embryo membrane.

In line with the experience of runt disease in mice, the
reaction does not occur with closely inbred chickens. If one
has access to such a line and tests blood from an adult bird
on chick embryos of the same stock, there are either no foci
or a very small number compared with the count obtained on
genetically distinct embryos. The influence of genetic factors
can be seen particularly clearly when two genes only are involved. In one experiment, cells from a cock (AA) were tested
on four of his own offspring in eggs laid by one hen with the
constitution AB. Two of the membranes had no foci whatever,
while the other two had 110 and 203 foci respectively; the
first two were clearly AA, the second pair AB.

The lesions are undoubtedly initiated by the white cells
of the blood and in all probability by lymphocytes only. The
number of foci produced by a known number of leukocytes
can therefore give quantitative information on the proportion
of cells capable of initiating the process. In round figures, one
lesion corresponds to about 10,000 lymphocytes.

There is evidence that the implanted cells multiply in the
embryo and retain at least some of their qualities. One can
carry on the phenomenon from one embryo to the next by
making a suspension of cells from the enlarged embryo spleen
and testing this on another chorioallantoic membrane. Numerous spots develop, though their size is smaller and more variable than those obtained directly from adult blood cells. In
our experience, this embryo-to-embryo passage fails after
three or four transfers.

Possibly the point of greatest interest is the speed with
which the reaction is initiated. The structure of the foci as

seen in sections made at 2, 3, and 4 days indicates that they must start their development within a few hours of the cells' being deposited on the membrane. Since cells from normal birds are used as inoculum, this must mean either that the cells are preadapted to react when they encounter a foreign antigen in the cells of the embryonic host or that the whole process of recognizing the foreign antigen and tooling up to produce antibody against it is completed within the isolated cell and in the space of a few hours. This finding is, we believe, very relevant to the current controversy between selective and instructive theories of immunity.

The last feature of the reaction which calls for comment is the way in which the opaque white foci develop on the chorioallantoic membrane. They take this form because of a massive proliferation of cells, mostly the embryo's own cells but in part cells that are descendants of those inoculated. Much still needs to be learned about the process, but in broad outline it appears that, when the adult immunologically competent cell meets the foreign antigen with which it can react, substances are produced which stimulate both foreign and adjacent host cells to proliferate. With more immunologically competent foreign cells and more host cells producing antigen for them to react with, the stage is set for a kind of vicious circle which soon leads to a close-packed mass of damaged cells. This is the opaque center of the developed focus.

7. The Clonal-Selection Theory of Immunity

Within the last 3 or 4 years, there has been something of a revolution in thinking about the basis of immunity. Until the Danish immunologist Jerne published his suggestion for a "natural-selection" theory of immunity in 1956, all immunologists were agreed in believing that the foreign material, the antigen, impressed its mark on the antibody-producing cells, compelling or instructing them to produce antibody with an appropriate complementary pattern that would give the best possible fit with the antigen. It was felt that we were dealing with something almost as definite as the relation between the pattern on the face of a coin and that on the die which stamped it. The metaphor was often used that the antigen was incorporated in the cell as a die which stamped its pattern on the gamma globulin as it was being produced by the cell.

Jerne in essence said, How do we know that the antigen

instructs the cells to produce such and such an antibody? Could it not be that they produce spontaneously a wide variety of potential antibodies and that when an antigen enters the body it is met by one of these natural antibody molecules carrying an appropriate pattern? As a result of this meeting a call goes out for the production of more of this particular sort of natural antibody.

This idea acted as a stimulus to several of those interested in immunological theories and in 1957 both Talmage and Burnet published accounts of ways in which a selection theory could be developed to account for many of the difficulties which had not been resolved by older theories. For obvious enough reasons, I shall discuss these selection theories mainly in terms of the so-called clonal-selection theory for which I was responsible. It is the simplest self-consistent theory, and, because it is so inherently simple, it is probably wrong. As yet, however, no decisive evidence against it has been produced and it is a good rule not to complicate assumptions until absolutely necessary. Occam's razor is still a useful tool.

The clonal-selection theory is a generalization about a wide range of biological phenomena and suffers from the inherent weakness of all biological generalizations. It can be only a partial picture of reality and its function is the purely provisional one of making it easier to think effectively about a complex mass of observational and experimental data. Perhaps because of the inescapable relation of the thinker, himself an organism and a product of evolution, to the things he is thinking about, biological understanding will always have a specially provisional quality. In many ways it is ridiculous to attempt generalization about somatic cells when we know almost nothing significant about the process of cellular differentiation. Yet from other points of view theoretical formulation in the light of current knowledge must always be going on. Neither education nor practical action in scientific fields is possible without a working set of provisional generalizations, and progress in research needs a constant emergence of working hypotheses to be put to the test of experiment.

It is the main — strictly speaking, the only — virtue of a good generalization that it can provoke scientists to design experiments which can prove it wrong. No experiment or observation can ever prove that it is right. The history of any scientific theory or generalization must from the nature of science be a continuing rearguard action. As one or other aspect is proved to be wrong or incomplete, it must be modified to fit the new facts until eventually it is changed almost out of recognition or is discarded. If in the process it has accelerated the development of a field of knowledge, it has more than fulfilled its function.

The essence of the clonal-selection theory is that immunity and antibody production are functions of clones of mesenchymal cells. Each clone is characterized by the ability of its component cells to react immunologically with a very small number of antigenic determinants. The number may be two in all instances, but one, three, or four are also conceivable. The nature of an antigenic determinant as a limited chemical configuration on the surface of an antigenic macromolecule or particle has already been discussed (Chapter 5). A cell is immunologically competent because it carries on its surface a receptor — a pattern analogous to antibody and perhaps legitimately pictured as cell-bound antibody — which allows it to react with a given antigenic determinant. It is immaterial for the moment whether it has any other types of receptor. Contact with the right antigenic configuration acts as a trigger to action and it is the essence of a clonal theory that such stimulation plays a major part in determining the observed changes in type and numbers of the mesenchymal cells of the body.

The trigger of immunological contact is believed to provoke actions which, depending on many associated factors, may take one or other of several forms. The cells may be killed or damaged, with release of cell-damaging or stimulating products; they may be stimulated to proliferate, with or without change of morphological type; or they may be converted to the plasma-cell form, with its capacity for active synthesis and liberation of antibody. Which particular reaction ensues will depend essentially on the physiological state of the cell and the nature of the internal environment to which it is exposed after stimulation.

For reasons that have already been discussed, the adult body contains only cells bearing immunological patterns which correspond to antigenic determinants that are *not* represented among the body's own constituents.

If we accept the theory, we can assume that every lymphocyte, plasma cell, or macrophage in the body is labeled by its immunological reactivity. There may be of the order of 10,000 such labels, with each cell carrying an average of two. This would require the existence of 10^8 potential clones, each by hypothesis derived from one or a very small number of ancestral cells by somatic multiplication.

A majority of immunologists find it difficult to accept the hypothesis that 10^4 or more different patterns of reactivity can be produced during embryonic life without reference to the foreign antigenic determinants with which they are "designed" to react. This response is perhaps more intuitive than logical. After all, we know that in the course of embryonic development an extraordinary range of information — probably many million "bits" — is interpreted into bodily structure and function. There is no intrinsic need for us to hesitate to ask for another 10,000 specifications to be carried in the genetic information of the fertilized egg. There are also at least three ways in which we can imagine the origin of those 10,000 patterns:

(1) It may be laid down in the genetic structure that in the course of development the whole 10,000 patterns will be produced at the appropriate time and in the appropriate tissue. In other words, we accept their appearance as part of the normal process of differentiation and ask no more about it.

(2) Somatic mutation is known to occur and it is also known that some regions of the genetic apparatus are more prone to mutation than others. If in ancestral mesenchymal cells that portion of the genetic mechanism responsible for specifying the pattern of antibody became for some period of embryonic life highly mutable, we could have the appearance of a very large series of random patterns that would provide the volume of antibody types that we need.

(3) It is a recent suggestion, arising from Szilard's ideas, that the available patterns are all based on the vast but by no means infinite range of chemical patterns that the cell can produce and manipulate with its enzymes. This is essentially a variant of the first alternative and would require too technical a discussion for its further elaboration.

The special need of selection theories for a large population with randomly determined characters on which selection can act makes us strongly favor the second alternative of transient high somatic mutability. None of the three suggestions is, however, necessarily correct, nor is the claim for the existence of 10,000 clones itself established. One can sympathize with those who ask why all this elaboration is necessary when the straightforward "instructive" theory is available. The answer is that it is needed to account for the phenomena described in Chapter 6 and concerned with the recognition of self. It is of particular significance that recognition as self can extend to substances or cells of different genetic origin which have been introduced into the body in embryonic or early postnatal life. Somehow we must find an explanation of how during embryonic life the body acquires or generates the information which allows it to differentiate immunologically between what is self and what is not self.

In attempting to describe the sort of process that will be needed to generate such information, it is, I believe, worth while developing an analogy with a more familiar type of information transfer — by words. To do so requires a certain amount of recapitulation and elaboration of the nature of the patterns which are mutually concerned in immunological reactions. There is good experimental evidence that the areas of interaction between the two giant molecules of a typical antigen and antibody are quite small. In each instance it seems likely that a configuration of two to five amino acid groupings or equivalent units is involved.

If it is true that around four amino acid units are responsible for each specific immune pattern, whether of antibody or of cell surface, we are again in a position to make use of the analogy between the 20 common biological amino acids and the letters of the alphabet (see Chapter 6). Each pattern could be represented by a four-letter combination, apqr for example. For simplicity we shall assume that all patterns are four-letter ones without discarding the possibility that some might be better represented by two-, three-, or five-letter groups. For an analogue of the random process which gives rise during embryonic life to the huge variety of potential patterns, we can imagine an electronic computer set to produce at random four-letter groups from a 26-letter alphabet. If 10^7 words are asked for, we should have a 99-percent probability of getting at least one example of every possible four-letter word. As an example of eight consecutive words we might find

  tres abcd apqr cxab ojbd *they* xpml *face*

Now suppose we have English-speakers watching the output and striking out all the English words, in this instance "they" and "face." In the final collection we have theoretically all the information required to construct all English four-letter words. Any combination which is not present is an English word. In the same way one-, two-, and three-letter words could be produced and similarly sorted out into English words, which are discarded, and non-English, which remain.

Our computer has another characteristic. Once the selection has been completed, all the remaining "words" are stored in the memory and when any combination is asked for it can be produced in unlimited numbers, but only if it is in the memory. No English will be produced. As I have indicated, an antibody or an antibody-producing cell carries a pattern which corresponds in a positive-negative complementary way with a rather small chemical configuration which could be represented reasonably by a four-letter combination, say APQR. The antibody or cell could then be indicated by the same letters in lower case to indicate that contact between APQR (antigen) and apqr (antibody or cell) will have a key-lock quality which can initiate a variety of physical or biological processes. There is sound analogy at least for believing that, if such contact between antigenic pattern and complementary cell takes place in embryonic life, the cell will be destroyed or, what amounts to the same thing, prevented from multiplying.

The clonal-selection theory assumes that this allows the same sort of generation of information as we obtained by having English-speakers strike out all the words they recognized. Pressing the analogy, we conceive that all the body's own components correspond to English two-, three-, or four-letter words, and to indicate how much information can be compressed into such simple material I have summarized the clonal-selection theory of immunity in the following collection of English words of four letters or less: "To know self from not self is a main need for life. In the womb it is laid down what is to be let live in the body. Self is what no cell dare act upon to harm; any cell that may harm self must die. What may come from air or soil the body will deal with as evil. A cell eats the germ for this is the best way to keep it from harm. Also any cell line made apt in the womb will when they meet the key unit grow fast if the dose of it is tiny but die if it is too much."

Whenever the molecular pattern corresponding to one of these words meets a cell carrying a complementary pattern (lower-case letters "the," "main," and so forth), contact is presumed to be lethal for the cell and eventually for all members of clones complementary to body components. By the time of birth all English (self) clones will have been eliminated.

Around the time of birth or hatching, the cells with which we have been concerned change their reactivity. Instead of leading to inhibition or destruction of the cell, contact with the corresponding antigen now is a stimulus to the cell to proliferate and produce antibody. Pattern APQR enters the body, perhaps as part of a not very dangerous bacterium. Sooner or later it meets cells of clones carrying apqr, which as a result are stimulated to multiply and to produce a population of antibody molecules which will play some part in hindering any harmful activities of the bacterium.

There is no need to describe what an antibody can do to a bacterium, or even to claim that antibody is the most important element in the body's defenses. In some cases, however, it is extremely effective, not only killing but also disintegrating the invader. Obviously there must be some way in which such destructive activities are directed only against foreign material or cells and not against the body's own components. In developing our analogy of English and not-English words, I hope that I have shown one reasonable way in which during embryonic life each one of us generates a fund of information which ensures that foreign material will be appropriately dealt with, while self material is unaffected.

This is the crux of the clonal-selection theory. If such information is generated, it must surely be in some such fashion as we have outlined; most of the other theories of immunity simply fail both to ask the question and to supply the answer.

A clonal-selection theory is primarily concerned with clones of cells and must name those cell types which are involved. In Chapter 5 an account was given of the probable interrelationships of stem cells, lymphocytes, plasma cells, and macrophages. In the clonal-selection theory it is assumed that a single clone, all members of which carry potential capacity to react with the same antigenic determinants, may contain a full range of mesenchymal types. Some, such as the red cell and the granulocyte, seem to have no capacity either for immunological reaction or for reversion to less specialized phases. If we are correct in ascribing the important activities to stem cell, lymphocyte, and plasma cell, and less important ones to macrophage, we can hardly avoid naming the lymphocyte as our chief vehicle of immunological information. It has all the necessary characters for such a role. In the first place, the cells must be mobile, moving to every part of the body that could conceivably be invaded by foreign material; they must be numerous, because by theory we may have to call on any one of perhaps 10^4 clones; and they must be capable of both rapid proliferation and rapid elimination if quick response is to be made to the emergencies of infection. There are about 10^{13} lymphocytes in the human body, of which less than 1 percent ($\pm$ 0.2 percent) are circulating in the blood. Their average life may be about 3 weeks, but there is much to suggest that some may live only a few hours, others the best part of a year. Modern work shows that they move constantly out of the blood into the tissues and back to the blood. They are always being produced and being destroyed. Lymphocytes are, in fact, more rapidly destroyed than any other cells in the body by such agents as x-rays and the cortisone group of drugs. They behave as if they were there to react quickly to some emergency situation.

The other point to be mentioned is the nature of the cell itself. Suppose we had to design a cell for this function of a repository of information — to be able to recognize a specific stimulus and thereupon to switch to proliferation and secretory activity as needed. Anyone with any knowledge of cytology will agree that the *work* of a functioning cell is carried out by the cytoplasm. The nucleus is there as a headquarters, not as a work force, a storehouse for the information needed to allow the replication of the cell and maintenance of cytoplasmic activity.

Clearly, if we want a cell with the qualities I have mentioned we should need one with a full store of genetic information and many potentialities, that is, a well-developed nucleus. But it would have no existing need for effector mechanisms in the cytoplasm. All that would be needed there would be the means to convey information to the nucleus — presumably surface receptors and the minimum of cytoplasm required for their maintenance.

This is actually a precise description of the small lymphocyte.

The clonal-selection theory can be elaborated in many ways, and by the use of reasonable *ad hoc* assumptions where necessary it can be made to cover all the established phenomena of immunity. It has also potentialities of further modification, for example, by admitting the possibility, now being widely looked for, of the transfer of genetic (and immuno-logical) information from one somatic cell to another. This is not the place to elaborate the theory indefinitely and we can probably provide the clearest over-all picture of how immunity develops according to this particular view by giving a circumstantial account in simplified terms of what happens in the young animal emerging from the sheltered intrauterine environment into the hazards of the external world. It must be emphasized that much of this account is outright specula-tion — but it will illustrate the implications of the clonal-selection approach.

The thymus is the organ in which mesenchymal cells, once their potential immunological label has been applied, con-centrate during embryonic life. These are cells which have not been inhibited prenatally and carry labels only for non-self antigenic determinants. If there are 5000 remaining pat-terns, these are produced at random and distributed in ran-dom pairs to the cells from which different clones derive. As soon, however, as bacteria appear in the bowel after birth, the opportunity and necessity for immunological re-action arises. When antigenic determinant A meets a cell of clone a, the cell is modified and stimulated to dedifferentiate and proliferate in spleen or lymph node to produce more lymphocytes of clone a but with a heightened reactivity. When these react again with antigen A, they are driven to proliferate more freely. If they lodge in a lymphoid follicle they initiate a germinal center, giving rise to more lympho-cytes. If they settle in other parts of spleen and lymph node, they will develop to plasma cells and produce antibody. It may be suggested as the best solution of a number of puzzling findings that cells returning to the thymus and there initiating lymphocyte production once again give rise to cells having only primary reactivity. As the individual ages and the thymus atrophies, it is only reasonable to believe that most of the circulating cells are of subclones which have developed secondary reactivity and are the products of multiplication in spleen and lymph nodes.

In the adult animal we can picture the existence of many stimulated clones corresponding to those antigens of which the animal has had experience plus a slowly diminishing complement of clones that have never undergone stimulation. Circulating antibody is a measure of the proportion of plasma cells in the clone; ability to respond in secondary fashion indicates the presence of stimulated subclones not necessarily in plasma-cell form. Perhaps it should be added that, whatever theory of antibody production and immunity is adopted, one would be compelled to visualize the distribution of the competent cells in very much the same fashion.

It would be a gratifying simplicity to find that all immunological reactivity was laid down prenatally and that no capacity to develop new patterns persisted into adult life. From general biological experience this seems most unlikely. Whatever the process by which new patterns emerge in prenatal life, it is probably still operative to a much reduced degree in postnatal life, though perhaps only in dedifferentiated rejuvenated cells. If this is the case, there must be in existence a control mechanism to prevent the emergence into activity of forbidden clones, that is, cells which react against components of the body. The simplest control mechanism to envisage is based on the assumption that, when an immunologically competent cell is stimulated by antigenic contact to initiate proliferation, it must pass through a dedifferentiated phase where fresh contact with antigen will result in its destruction or at least inability to go on to proliferation. In other words, any freely present antigenic pattern will inhibit proliferation of cells of the corresponding clones. This applies just as much to artificial circumstances when, for instance, very large amounts of foreign serum protein are given intravenously to a rabbit. The possibility of failure of this mechanism of control is discussed in relation to autoimmune disease in Chapter 11.

Genetic aspects of clonal selection

The clonal-selection hypothesis is concerned with qualities of body (somatic) cells by which groups of cells can maintain inheritable differences from one another over several or many cell generations. In essence we are concerned with the genetics of somatic cells. There is no evidence as yet that somatic cells can mate, or interchange genetic material in any other fashion. We are therefore precluded from the use of the standard methods of genetic analysis. There is, however, good reason to believe, on the basis both of the nature of cell duplication and of experimental observations, that within somatic cell populations mutations of the same general type as in germ cells must occur, and with the same order of frequency. In addition, we have to recognize that in the course of differentiation a whole series of controlled and directed changes in the genetic potentialities of the cells must take place. Of all the great territories of biology, this of differentiation is probably the least effectively explored.

There is no question that in an immunized animal there are cells which can give rise to descendant cells with definable immunological reactivity. Some means of transmitting the necessary genetic information must therefore be present in the clones concerned. It need not be carried in the nucleus or in DNA. Nevertheless, since this is the only way in which we *know* that genetic information can be carried in any organism larger than a virus, we have an a priori obligation to look first for such a mechanism.

Discussion, particularly with geneticists primarily interested in the behavior of microorganisms, has made it clear that there are many conceivable ways in which a selectionist theory of immunity could be expressed. We could assume that a diploid cell might have a pair of chromosomes each bearing a locus that controlled one antibody type pattern. Such cells might be able to make one antibody or two antibodies but not more. On the other hand, there is no a priori reason why there should not be the genetic information for three or ten different patterns in each cell, with some arrangement to ensure that not more than two examples were called into activity simultaneously. Any substantial increase in the number of potential immune patterns would, however, remove the most attractive feature of the clonal-selection hypothesis — its ability to account for self-recognition by the elimination of forbidden clones at the cellular level. There are undoubtedly ways by which one could imagine continuing inhibition of certain cellular potentialities without actual destruction of the cells concerned and still retain the essential features of clonal selection, namely, preadaptation, limited reactivity, and transmission of immunological memory through somatic-cell generations. Such possibilities, however, will come up for discussion only when the simple clonal-selection theory is proved to be inadequate.

There are other possibilities, in which the nuclear DNA mechanism is bypassed and the information located in the ribosomes (RNA) of the cytoplasm or in the RNA of the nucleus, perhaps in the nucleolus. If we accept that ribosomal protein-synthetic mechanisms once initiated by the nucleus are capable of continued activity and to some extent, at least, of self-replication, none of the facts of immunity rule out this possibility. It will be more convenient, however, to discuss this possibility when the other types of immunological theory are considered in the next chapter.

Perhaps the strongest reason for seeking a theory of anti-body production which does not make the antigen responsible for bringing the necessary information into the cell comes from modern work on the adaptive enzymes of bacteria. Enzymes and antibodies have much in common, and the observation that enzymes were often produced — it seemed *ab initio* — only after contact with the substrate offered a special reason for regarding antibodies as very closely related to such adaptive enzymes. It is now almost unanimously accepted that a bacterium can produce only such adaptive enzymes as its genetic make-up allows and that in many cases it can be shown that the action of the substrate or inducer is to release an inhibitor which normally keeps the enzyme-synthesizing machinery inactive. It has become a virtual dogma that recognizable differences in protein structure are produced by the sequence of information flow

$$DNA \rightarrow RNA \rightarrow protein,$$

and that in general one looks for the basic difference in genetic information that gives rise to protein differences in the coding of the DNA. It has become almost a Lamarckian heresy to believe that any meaningful inheritable change of structure can be impressed either on a protein or on any part of the genetic mechanism by the action of environmental factors. Increased frequency of random mutation or chromosomal damage can readily be produced by radiation and by such chemicals as nitrogen-mustard gas, but the changes in the organism that result from mutations are quite irrelevant to the nature of the agent that produces them. Throughout the history of biology we have seen the progressive disproof of theories by which the environment generated organisms or enforced changes on them. The sun does not breed maggots in a dead dog nor does Nile mud generate swallows. Bacteria do not arise by spontaneous generation nor herpes virus by the action of wind and sunshine on the lips. It is sound dogma that inheritable change can be induced only by modification or transfer of genetic information and must be discussed in genetic terms. If antibody production and immunological specificity are characters that can be passed along a line of cells, we can expect them to arise by mutation, by differentiation, or by transfer from some other genetic system but not by a direct impact of a pattern from the environment on the cell.

8. The Other Theories of Immunity

In the course of much discussion in most parts of the world during the period 1958–1960, I gained the general impression that most chemists and immunologists strongly favored the orthodox view of antibody production as something whose specificity is directly shaped by the antigen, while those geneticists who were interested in the general problem tended to favor the clonal-selection ideas or some modification thereof.

It is very necessary, therefore, to present as attractively as possible the orthodox theoretical approach as it has been developed since 1937 by Landsteiner, Mudd, Haurowitz, Pauling, and Karush. In the very early days of immunology Ehrlich's ideas, as expressed in the side-chain theory of antibody production, were selectionist in character. The antibody represented an overproduction of something preexistent (and therefore genetically determined) in the cell. Landsteiner, interested in the chemistry of immunity, found that he could produce antibodies reacting with synthetic compounds like arsanilic acid which could never have existed in nature. He saw no escape from the assumption that the foreign antigen impressed a complementary pattern on the globulin as it was being produced by the cell. Pauling in 1940 held that this view could be elaborated in such a fashion that no violence was done to current concepts of protein structure and behavior and has since strongly upheld its validity.

In its modern form, Pauling's theory holds that gamma globulin as primarily synthesized in the form of polypeptide chains has no immunological character. This it is endowed with by the processes of secondary and tertiary folding that convert a long tenuous filament into a globular or spindle-shaped antibody molecule. Karush pictures the primary folding as producing a plastic entity (in the sense that many different configurations are all thermodynamically equally probable) which can be pushed into a sterically complementary shape by physical contact with the antigenic determinant. When the molding process is completed, the folded chain can be stabilized into a permanent structure by the closing of –S–S– or hydrogen bonds between adjacent segments. Thereafter the antigenic template is released, perhaps then to be applied to another aspect of the forming macromolecule. As long as the antigen remains in the cell, it can continue to serve as the template for the final folding that confers its specific character on the antibody. An antigenic determinant is a very small chemical structure and a little calculation shows that one antigenic determinant for every lymphoid cell in the human body would require less than a microgram (0.000001 gm), so that there is no way of ever proving that antigen is *not* present in an antibody-producing cell.

There are considerable objections at the chemical level to this hypothesis, at least in Karush's form. All that we know of the structure of those small proteins and polypeptides which have been completely characterized indicates that the

–S–S– connections between peptide chains are by no means random. There are only a limited number of ways in which intramolecular bonds can develop and there appears to be a considerable body of opinion that, given the size and sequence of a polypeptide chain and the general physical quality of the environment into which it is liberated, the way in which its secondary and tertiary folding will develop is predetermined.

Recent work indicates that rabbit antibody can be split into three roughly equal fragments, two of which have the characteristic signature of antibody in being able to combine with antigen though not to precipitate with it. The third is a very easily crystallized protein that is a good *antigen* but has no activity whatever as an antibody. It seems likely that several different synthetic processes converge to produce a single antibody molecule and it may well be that only one of these is specially concerned with the immunological pattern of the antibody. There is still too little known about the details of intracellular processes to allow us to exclude categorically the possibility that in some way a fragment of antigen might be built into a protein-synthetic mechanism, or some sort of "geno-copy" produced to allow its passage from cell to cell. All one can say is that the general development of thought on the processes which allow the expression of genetic information in the form of functional protein seems to point right away from this type of approach.

There is at least one way by which a theory which claims that antibody specificity is wholly a function of the secondary or tertiary structure of the globulin molecule could be proved wrong. This would be to show that several antibodies made in the same species of animal against antigens of similar type each had a different and characteristic primary structure. When, as in the present instance, we want to determine whether or not two or more proteins are chemically identical, it is not always necessary to obtain the complete chemical structure of each protein. There is a technique, known in laboratory slang as "fingerprinting," which can often give us the necessary information. Enough is now known about the way various purified enzymes break down protein molecules for the biochemist to prepare appropriate digests of the proteins he is interested in, which contain mixtures of various protein fragments each composed of a few amino acids linked into small peptides. By appropriate techniques of paper chromatography and electrophoresis, a complex pattern of blots and smudges on a sheet of filter paper is obtained for the various digests. These are the fingerprints which can allow us to recognize differences between superficially similar proteins. The first great achievement by this technique was the demonstration by Ingram that the hemoglobin from persons with sickle-cell disease of the blood differed from normal hemoglobin; one amino acid is replaced by another at a single position in one of the two primary protein units which make up the hemoglobin molecule.

Obviously this was a technique that should be applied to the antibody problem, and the first report of experiments on these lines appeared in 1960. Gitlin found, in fact, that there were clear-cut differences among antibodies to be shown by the fingerprint method. The antibodies he used were prepared by immunizing rabbits with pure polysaccharide antigens from three types of *Pneumococci* and isolated from the serum by union with the corresponding antigen. On enzyme digestion each antibody gave its own distinctive fingerprint pattern.

There are many technical difficulties in such work and it is probably wise to reserve final judgment until Gitlin's results have been confirmed by others. If there are differences in the primary structure of antibody globulins related to the functional specificity of the antibodies, this is obviously the most important discovery yet made in the chemistry of immunity. It would clearly abolish the current form of the instructive theory of antibody production. If each type of antibody has a characteristic primary sequence of amino acids, then the information required for its assembly must be carried in the genetic mechanism of the cell producing it. Any instructive theory is then directly faced with the necessity of claiming a specific modification of genetic structure by an environmental stimulus in the form of an antigenic determinant. This is virtually impossible to conceive on any currently accepted view of the process by which genetic information is stored.

A special disadvantage of "instructive" theories, that is, theories which assume that the pattern of the antigen directly determines the pattern of the antibody produced, is their failure to offer any suggestion why self components are nonantigenic.

Elective or selective theories, by which an antigen finds a preexistent pattern with which it can react and as a result initiates various types of cellular activity, can more readily be manipulated to explain the phenomena of self-recognition and tolerance. It is by no means necessary, however, that they should be cast in the form of the clonal-selection theory.

However unlikely it sounds, there is no real reason for denying the possibility that each lymphoid cell may contain 10,000 specific receptors, one tuned to each of all the possible antigenic patterns. It is also just conceivable that during embryonic life 5000 or some such number of receptors in each cell are eliminated or inhibited by contact with body patterns, so providing at a subcellular level the same sort of explanation of tolerance that is given at the cellular level by the clonal-selection approach.

This may all be true, but the hypothesis is rather unattractive simply because there is no clear operational approach to differentiating it from the instructive-type theories. There is no way of distinguishing between a cell that can make thousands of different antibodies because it has preexistent patterns ready for eventual stimulus and another which does this by using the antigen itself as a mold or template.

The argument most frequently raised against selection theories of immunity is the finding by Landsteiner and others that antibodies could be produced against quite unphysiological substances such as arsanilic acids. This is, in fact, quite irrelevant. The antibody has been produced and we must assume that, like every other antibody, it unites with the arsanilic acid determinant because of a certain localized configuration of amino acid residues. This configuration exists and must therefore be one of the complete range of possible patterns which, according to clonal-selection theory, can be produced by some random process during early development of the embryo. Of those which are not eliminated during embryonic life as corresponding to self patterns, there are just as likely to be patterns corresponding to potential unbiological antigenic determinants as to determinants of more familiar sort. Since *all* are produced not from models but at random, the argument loses all its force.

Clonal selection, in which all phenomena are considered at the cellular instead of the subcellular level, is more amenable to experimental test. It is disconcerting, however, to find that up to the present no experiments have been reported which can be regarded as providing a crucial test.

It would be ideal if it were possible to obtain a group of immune cells and grow each separately in tissue culture to give actual clones of cells which could then be tested for immunological activity. Unfortunately, it is the usual finding that when functional cells from an adult individual are grown in tissue culture they will grow freely only if, after undergoing mutation or some equivalent change, they lose all their normal function and become dedifferentiated multiplying cells with no other activity than proliferation. So far no group skilled in both immunology and tissue culture has made a deliberate attack on this problem. There are a number of ways in which it could be approached, but the simplest would be to start by immunizing a pure-strain mouse with some standard antigen. From a stimulated lymph node a dozen single-cell clones would be developed in the hope that one or two of them would be of immunologically effective cells. To test this, part of the clone would be returned to mice of the same strain which had been treated with x-rays to make them more receptive of the cells. It is most unlikely that the cells would forthwith make antibody, but their competence could be tested by injecting the mice with the antigen and seeing whether a primary or a secondary immune response resulted. A secondary response would be positive evidence that the character of the cells had been maintained. Once a positive finding had been obtained, the study could be elaborated in various directions.

Even if the result indicated that a thoroughly active clone of cells could retain its characteristic activity indefinitely, this would not establish that the clonal-selection theory was correct. It would merely show that, once a line of immune cells had developed, the immune character could be passed on by some form of genetic mechanism. The problem is really how the *first* stage of immunization takes place. Here we come against a major difficulty: when we are dealing with an antigen that the animal has never previously encountered, the first response is slow and small. This is reasonable on any theory, but it makes it extraordinarily difficult to devise experiments to decide between the various alternatives.

There are bacterial extracts which when given to rabbits without antibody against the antigens will rapidly provoke antibody production. Although there is still some considerable doubt about how much antibody a single cell will produce, the results point strongly toward the conclusion that there is a significantly large proportion of lymphoid cells in the rabbit which can be forced to respond to contact with the antigen by antibody production. Either they respond directly in the fashion claimed by instructive theories or there is a much larger proportion of cells preadapted to produce this type of bacterial antibody than the 0.01 percent or less postulated by simple clonal selection. The difficulty in interpretation here is one that plagues all immunological experiments with the usual laboratory animals — their past experience of bacterial infection, particularly in the intestine.

Immediately after birth foreign antigenic material begins to seep into the body in the form of a wide variety of bacterial and protozoal components. There are probably very important processes at work during the first few days of life, when the system of cells prepared for immunological activity is still completely immature. Observation of animals reared in the complete absence of bacteria indicates that the maturation of the system is largely due to the normal contact with bacterial antigens in the intestine. No one has yet made a real appreciation of what actually happens in this critical period, in terms of cellular and immunological events. It is impossible to claim that it is early experience of this sort that makes a rabbit's lymphoid cells so responsive to a variety of bacterial antigens, but until the early experience is understood we shall find it difficult to devise adequate experimental tests on the nature of the primary action of foreign antigens.

There is one experiment which is technically conceivable by which the clonal-selection theory could be decisively disproved. This is to obtain a pure clone in tissue culture of mesenchymal cells, again from a mouse of a pure-line strain, and build up an adequate supply of descendant cells. We now choose six standard antigens whose corresponding antibodies are known not to be present in normal mouse serum. Each is used to treat a portion of the stock of pure clone cells in the test tube. The cells are then washed to get rid of most of the antigen and injected into mice of the original strain and preferably treated with x-rays 24 hours before the injection. If a week later the mice were found to be producing antibody corresponding to two or more of the antigens used, we should be compelled to discard the theory in any usefully simple form.

The only escape would be to postulate a rate of random mutation of pattern as high as that assumed to occur in early embryonic life. If it were possible to obtain antibody production with very small numbers of cells, even this remote possibility could probably be excluded.

If a pure clone of cells could be made to produce antibody of more than one type in the test tube, this would be even more decisive, but no experiments of this type have been described and success would seem to be extremely unlikely.

The weight of these two chapters on theories of immunity falls on the side of selective as against instructive theories — not, I hope, simply because I have personally sponsored one of the selective theories. From the standpoint of the philosophy of biology, the selective approach seems much more attractive. Nevertheless, one should be very ready to admit that from the pragmatic approach of the user of immunological methods the instructive view is the more convenient. When we want a serum that will react with a given protein and make the appropriate inoculations of a group of rabbits, we can hardly avoid picturing the process as a straightforward instructive one. At the level of the immunochemist, everything proceeds *as if* antigenic determinants impressed their complementary patterns on the globulin, so transforming it into the desired reagent. It is only at a more sophisticated level that we begin to wonder why rabbit albumin is not antigenic in the rabbit, and recognize that something less straightforward is required.

9. The Nonmedical Applications of Immunology

Immunology, like all the other biological sciences, grew out of medicine but has come to have many applications in other than medical contexts. So far we have been concerned with the basic phenomena and their theoretical interpretation. Now we can concentrate on the use to be made of immunological techniques, and in subsequent chapters on some of the immunological problems in human medicine.

Chemically speaking, a protein is an unmanageably complex and rather featureless compound when examined by orthodox chemical techniques. The only chemically interesting proteins are those which are small, very constant in composition, and readily crystallized. In a protein like insulin it is possible to apply refined chemical methods to give the complete structure of the molecule. Similar success is in sight for pancreatic ribonuclease, but at a very heavy cost in time and effort.

In general, a protein interests a biologist only in terms of what it does, and very often one can find this out only by elaborate biological experiments. For the chemist interested in proteins there are very obvious advantages if the protein has some functional activity which can be measured apart from any living system, in some more or less complicated test tube. Enzymes and antibodies provide many suitable examples. It is possible to estimate accurately extremely small amounts of enzyme protein by measuring the rate at which it acts on the appropriate substrate, and most modern studies on the synthesis of protein make use of a method of this sort.

In biochemical research we are almost always dealing with complex mixtures of proteins which require much elaborate manipulation to extract one particular component in pure form. If, however, the component we are interested in has a "label" attached, one can recognize and measure it without interference by the other proteins present — an enormous technical simplification. As I have indicated in earlier chapters, the synthesis of antibody is too controversial a matter for antibody to be a suitable labeled protein for basic studies; but as long as its special qualities are understood, its label makes antibody very valuable for the analysis of many physiological problems.

Another application of this principle of labeling a protein or other biological molecule is to use an appropriate antibody to "recognize" the substance we are interested in. Such methods have very wide application throughout the biological sciences.

We may have the problem of purifying a protein with some important functional character, diphtheria toxin, for example. This is known to be an excellent antigen, reacting as we have described with antitoxin in a variety of ways. One method is to allow antitoxin and toxin both to diffuse into an agar jelly from two sources a few centimeters apart. Where antigen and antibody meet and react, an opaque line of precipitate forms. If we are concerned with a pure antigen and its antiserum, there will be a single well-defined line. If, however, the material we are using as antigen contains several immunologically active components, their interactions with different sets of antibody molecules in the antiserum will almost certainly produce multiple lines of precipitation. This can give important guidance during the process of physical or chemical purification.

Another relatively common type of problem in enzyme chemistry is to know whether two enzymes which appear to be functionally similar have the same chemical structure. There was a classic problem, for instance, to find whether the enzyme β-galactosidase produced as an adaptive enzyme, that is, on demand when its substrate was present, was the same as a similarly active enzyme that was produced in the absence of substrate by a mutant of the same bacterium. Immunologically the two enzyme proteins behaved identically. The enzyme penicillinase that makes some staphylococci resistant to treatment with penicillin is immunologically similar in all such strains but is quite different from the penicillinase produced by another type of bacterium (*Bacillus cereus*).

There is no limit to the number of such applications. The essential feature is that we should have available an antiserum which will react only with the substance we are interested in and not with any other substances that are present or may be present in the various fluids, extracts, and so forth that are being studied. Sometimes it will need careful study of all aspects of the system before a satisfactory reagent can be produced. This holds particularly when we are trying to follow the behavior of a protein that is always to be found in association with other rather closely related proteins. Suppose, for instance, that we wished to find how rapidly a dose of horse serum injected into a human being was eliminated from the body. One way would be to take samples of blood from the subject at appropriate times after the injection and separate the serum. This could then be tested with an anti-serum made by injecting rabbits with horse serum. The amount of precipitate could be expected to give a measure of the amount of horse protein still present. In fact, a much more elaborate procedure would be needed. The horse serum would first be fractionated to obtain the particular component that is relevant to the purpose of the experiment and rabbits would be immunized with this. The serum so obtained would probably also react to a lesser extent with the similar fraction in human serum and before it could be used it would need to be treated ("absorbed") with human serum to remove this deceptive activity.

Sometimes a different method can be used to obtain the same sort of immune serum with sharply restricted activity. Baby rabbits are injected with, in this case, the human pro-tein to render them unresponsive or tolerant. Later they are injected with the horse protein and respond only to those aspects of the protein which differ from both the correspond-ing rabbit and human proteins.

Epidemiological and forensic applications

Blood, when it is found anywhere but in the veins of the man or animal to whom it belongs, is liable to be associated with important practical problems. In all sorts of circum-stances it may become necessary to identify the source of the blood: is it animal or human, and if human from whom?

A good example is the method used to determine the nature of the blood present in an engorged mosquito. This is a rou-tine part of the preliminary work needed before an antimalarial campaign can be initiated. The food preferences of the local malaria-carrying mosquitoes will often provide very helpful clues to the best methods of eliminating them. The technique is to crush each engorged mosquito on a little strip of filter paper, which soaks up the blood. Later an extract is made from the filter paper and tested against a battery of antisera appropriately absorbed to give antibodies specific for blood proteins of each of the species that are likely to be important in the country concerned.

Similar methods can be applied to any other type of blood-feeding animal, always provided that the meal can be obtained for testing before the process of digestion has proceeded too far.

The amount of information that can be obtained from blood-stained knives, clothes, and the rest, is well known to every reader of detective stories. Basically the same methods are used and if the material is reasonably fresh and in adequate amount tests of human blood for its blood groups can often add further information.

Practical immunology has a wide variety of other legal and forensic applications. If it is a legal requirement that hamburger meat shall be beef only, almost the only way of ensuring that a given sample contains no cheaper horse, whale, or kangaroo meat is to use appropriate immunological tests. Other types of mislabeling or substitution can be similarly detected.

In Chapter 6 and elsewhere we have discussed some of the genetic aspects of immunology. The chemical structure of every cell in the body is specified in detail in that enormous "library" of chemical information that is compressed into the minute nucleus of the fertilized egg. An antigen is a protein or other large molecule which differs in one or more regions of its structure from any substance of generally similar character in the animal being immunized. The differences are necessarily chemical and like every other aspect of the protein are genetically controlled. So if two related animals which can be hybridized to produce fertile offspring produce antigenically different cells or cell products, these differences can usually be used as direct indicators of genetic constitution. In human beings, the ABO blood groups are the best-known immunological "markers" of this sort, but any of the other blood groups can be used equally well. We know more about red-blood-cell antigens than about any other types of human antigens, simply because red-cell antibodies are very easily demonstrated by an agglutination technique and because of the great importance of avoiding immunological reactions in the course of blood transfusion. If the need and the techniques applied to other proteins and polysaccharides, similar genetically based complexities would undoubtedly emerge.

So it comes about that immunological methods have been applied to a large range of problems in what we can call "relationships." The general nature of human blood groups was described in Chapter 4 but there is still something to be said about their application to the problem of relationship, more specifically to problems of paternity. There are now a large number of blood-group systems, the ABO system, the Rh or CDE system, the MN system, and so on. As each system was discovered, the first step was to work out the nature of the inheritance of the various groups within the system. In the ABO group we know that an O individual has the genotype OO, and an AB individual must have the genotype AB, but A or B individuals can be either homozygous AA, BB, or heterozygous AO, BO. On this basis there are simple rules about what certain matings can give to their offspring and what they cannot. If a child of an O mother is group A, then the father is certainly not group O or group B.

Table 6 shows what could be expected from all possible matings in this system and tables similar in principle could be prepared for each of the other systems. A full blood examination of mother, child, and reputed father will nowadays almost always clarify the position. If in each system the child's group is one of the "possibles," it becomes virtually certain that the reputed father is the real father. If the child is illegitimate, there is only a very small probability that no discrepancy in the blood groups will be found.

Table 6. The rules of inheritance of the ABO blood groups as applied to paternity tests.

Mating	Possible	Impossible
O × O	O	A, B, AB
O × A	O, A	B, AB
O × B	O, B	A, AB
O × AB	A, B	O, AB
A × A	A, O	B, AB
A × B	O, A, B, AB	—
A × AB	A, B, AB	O
B × B	B, O	A, AB
B × AB	A, B, AB	O
AB × AB	A, B, AB	O

The same general approach can be made in cases of disputed paternity in stud cattle, though here the method of testing is more elaborate and less readily available.

The establishment of paternity is a matter of small-scale genetics. The immunological comparison of races and species can also be fruitful and we have already referred to the use that has been made of blood-group statistics by anthropologists in tracing race movements and relationships. Even wider relationships have been studied and a classical piece of pioneer immunology was Nuttall's study of "blood relationships" using precipitation of sera of different species by antibody produced against one of them. In general there is a reasonable correlation between cross-reactions shown immunologically and the degree of zoological relationship assessed by other criteria. If an antihorse serum is made in a rabbit, such antibody will react strongly with horse and donkey serum, less strongly with ox serum, and probably not at all with mouse or human serum. Such tests can be refined and made as quantitative as is desired by selecting a specific serum protein, albumin for example, for all tests and estimating the weight of antigen precipitated by a standard amount of antibody.

One of the most important tasks of immunochemistry in the near future is to compare the immunological reactions and the chemical structures of a range of functionally similar proteins from different species. At the present time, insulin is the only protein for which this information is available and insulin is a notoriously poor antigen. Nevertheless, there is a detectable immunological difference between beef and pork insulin which seems to be related to a single region of the molecule, the amino acid residues 8, 9, and 10 on the A chain. Theoretically, immunological analysis is a chemical analysis on a differential basis. We have a species, usually a rabbit, which serves as the producer of antibody, and as antigens we have a functionally similar protein from two different species. Purified bovine (BSA) and human (HSA) serum albumin may be taken as examples in view of the large amount of work which has been done on just this system. Immunologically, we are concerned essentially with the differences between rabbit serum albumin, RSA, and BSA on the one hand and HSA on the other. The main features of the reactions to be expected can be symbolized as in Table 7. Here we assume that there are nine antigenically significant groups, of which

Table 7. To illustrate the differential character of immunological
analysis of two proteins using rabbit antisera.

Protein *	Potential antigenic determinants	Antibody	Absorbed antibody
RSA	A B C D E F G H R		
BSA	A B C D E F J K V	j k v	v
HSA	A B C D E J K W Y	j k w y	w y

* RSA, rabbit serum albumin; BSA, bovine serum albumin; HSA, human serum albumin.

five are common to all and are therefore immunologically inert. The rabbit antibody contains the components shown, and when this is cross-absorbed with the heterologous antigen the antibody components shown in the final column are left. If this is a true interpretation of the facts, it demonstrates clearly the differential character of the immunological analysis. Obviously it would be of the greatest interest if the symbols could be interpreted in terms of known chemical configurations. When this can be done we shall be in a much stronger position to see the full significance of the genetic relationships which can be recognized by immunological tests.

The classification of microorganisms

One of the most important practical uses of the principles of immunology is for the classification of microorganisms. Immunology grew out of the study of infectious disease and it was very natural that physicians working in bacteriological laboratories should classify microbes according to their power to immunize. If we have three cultures of disease-producing bacteria, A, B, and C, and we find that after infection with A an animal is immune to A and C, but after being infected with B resists a new infection with B but is fully sensitive to A and

C, then we are obviously going to put A and C in one species and B in another. So first of all disease-producing bacteria and then viruses were divided into species or types by whatever immunological technique appeared to be most relevant and convenient. Where methods of artificial immunization had been developed, it was obviously important to include in the vaccine all the "types" which were responsible for any significant proportion of the disease in question. The Salk vaccine against polio, for example, contains three immunological types of polio virus.

The same principles are applicable to other microorganisms, irrespective of whether they are responsible for disease or not. Any systematic study of a group of bacteria will always include a division into "serological types" on the basis of agglutination by antisera made in rabbits. Two cultures will be accepted as of the same type if the antiserum against one is equally active in agglutinating the other and if absorption of the serum with either removes all action against both. Between complete identity and absence of any cross reaction whatever, there are many intermediate degrees. The finer analysis of bacterial relationships by serological techniques has been of great practical and theoretical importance, especially in sorting out the great group of bacteria (*Salmonella*) responsible for intestinal infections of various sorts, from typhoid fever to food poisoning. It would be inappropriate, however, to elaborate on this topic here.

Two other examples unrelated to disease may be mentioned. The protozoon *Paramecium* has been extensively used as an object of experimental study. It swims actively by means of rows of cilia and if these short vibrating threads are damaged the organism becomes immobile. If rabbits are injected with a pure culture of *Paramecium*, they develop an antibody which will immobilize a protozoon of the corresponding culture but not necessarily an animal from an unrelated culture. This provides a principle for classifying races of *Paramecium* and has also led Sonneborn to the important discovery that a given race of *Paramecium* can by various means be forced to take on one or other of seven immunological phases. This is not mutation but a switch among a limited number of predetermined patterns.

The second example concerns the bacterial viruses, bacteriophages. These minute parasites of bacteria are essentially composed of a mass of nucleic acid (DNA) surrounded by a protein capsule plus a complex tail with several protein constituents including fine filaments which are responsible for anchoring the virus to the wall of the bacterium that it attacks. There are antigenically active groups in each of these proteins, but the most commonly studied action of an antiserum is on the power of the virus to infect bacteria. The antibody concerned is directed against the tail filaments. If they are coated and clogged with antibody, they cannot spread out and attach to the bacterial wall and the virus is rendered harmless.

From this an excellent method of classifying bacterial viruses can be elaborated. As far as work has gone, it appears that the relationships so established correspond to the results obtained by hybridizing phages. Among mammals and birds, a species may be defined approximately as comprising individuals among which mating will give rise to fertile offspring. If we applied the same rule to bacterial viruses, the species so defined would correspond to the groups obtained by the immunological method.

10. Medical Applications of Immunology

For most people the justification for medical research is its contribution toward human well-being. Always the aim of medical science and practice has been to provide for all human beings the greatest measure of health and length of life that is allowed by their inheritance. Almost suddenly we have begun to realize that our success in this objective has raised an acute and urgent problem of world overpopulation which will certainly provide the most important social and political problems of the next 50 years. There are well-informed optimists who believe that by the wholehearted application of science to the full exploitation of the current resources of this planet up to 10,000 million people could be supported. This could give time for the development of the acceptance of birth control as a universal social obligation. The equally well-informed pessimists see no reason to draw from human history any assurance that a sane solution will be reached.

It is a pity that the modern scientist cannot recapture the old naïve faith that success in his undertakings could only be of unalloyed benefit to his fellows. It is a pity because the control of infectious disease by environmental control, by immunization, and by antimicrobial drugs has been something good enough to be proud of. The problems of preventing infectious disease have nearly all been solved in principle. Their application clearly requires only the well-directed expenditure of money and effort plus education and a rising standard of living in the regions in which infectious disease is still an important cause of death. There will always be need for detailed study and *ad hoc* research in dealing with these practical measures. Fundamental research in the field of infectious disease is nowadays concerned not so much with devising means of controlling infection but in seeking an understanding of the means which have proved effective.

The various applications of immunology have directly or indirectly played a great part in the progressive elimination of infectious disease. This has been the main impact of immunology on medicine in the past. In the future we can expect greater emphasis to be placed on the guidance modern immunology can give in avoiding the troubles associated with pregnancy, blood transfusion, and tissue transplantation, and in possible extensions of tissue-grafting procedures between different individuals. Even more important is the need to understand and if possible prevent and cure the important human diseases in which the immune mechanisms are functioning unhelpfully or have even set going a damaging or lethal attack on the body's own tissues. Rather closely related to these immunological diseases are some of the drug sensitivities that have appeared in rather disquieting numbers as a result of the flood of new and potent drugs that have been introduced into medicine in the last 30 years.

In this chapter we shall discuss the applications of immunology to medical and surgical procedures and in the following two chapters the allergic and autoimmune diseases.

Immunization against infectious disease

It is our pride that in a civilized country the only infectious diseases from which anyone is likely to suffer are either trivial or easily cured by available drugs. The diseases that killed in the past have in one way or another been rendered impotent and in the process general principles of control have been developed which should be applicable to any unexpected emergence of infectious disease in the future. Where a disease is easily recognizable either clinically or by convenient laboratory tests and produces very few subclinical cases (that is, invisible asymptomatic infections), it will usually be possible to stamp it out completely, provided the community is willing to submit to the inconvenience of any administrative action necessary. In Australia we have no smallpox, yellow fever, or rabies, no malaria or sleeping sickness, no typhus, no cholera or plague. These have either failed to enter or have been eliminated in one way or another after each entry into the country and are currently kept out by quarantine. If it is a practicable measure to eliminate an infection completely — whether affecting human beings or domestic animals — this is by far the most satisfactory solution.

Where this is impossible, there are two other approaches. If the infection cannot be eradicated because of its wide dissemination in wild animals or birds, it is often possible by simple measures to make human infection very rare. Mosquito control will almost eliminate human cases of virus encephalitis; simple precautions will protect against psittacosis, rabies, and tularemia. It is particularly in the human diseases spread from person to person that the approach by immunization is needed. Many of the infections of this group are predominantly subclinical. Entry and multiplication of the microorganism in the body will often produce no symptoms, or such trivial ones that a definite diagnosis can be made only when laboratory tests are applied. Diphtheria and polio are the prototypes of such diseases and provide, of course, the outstanding examples of successful immunization. In general the aim of artificial immunization is to provide a means that will produce the same degree of immunity as a subclinical attack of the disease, but without the associated risk. In regions like Australia, North America, and Western Europe, the standard childhood immunizations are against diphtheria, whooping cough, tetanus, and polio. Smallpox vaccination persists largely because of the advantage of having the active primary reaction in infancy rather than in adult life.

For travel in the tropics or from the tropics, immunization against smallpox and yellow fever is mandatory and in many regions vaccination against typhoid fever and cholera is advisable, and sometimes compulsory. In military forces circumstances often require immunization against typhus fever and against the main respiratory infections — influenza A and B and Adenoviruses 3 and 7 at the present time.

In earlier chapters a good deal has been said incidentally about some of the practical immunization procedures, especially those directed against diphtheria and polio. Here we are concerned not with practical details of age, dose, route of inoculation, and the like, but with the processes by which, following the prescribed injections, real protection is obtained. Vaccination against smallpox is particularly instructive and there are some aspects of some of the other common immunizations that are worth mentioning.

Immunization against smallpox by inoculation of the skin with virus derived from a related disease of the cow (*vacca*) was not only the first attempt at artificial immunization but gave the generic name, vaccination, used for many such procedures. The vaccine lymph now used is a suspension of living virus which *should* be a lineal descendant of the virus used by Jenner at the beginning of the 19th century. It is, however, not the same as the cowpox viruses now found in Britain, and many virologists think that it may be a derivative of human smallpox picked up in arm-to-arm vaccination in the early 19th century. In the last 2 or 3 years it has been shown that hybrids can be rather readily produced among viruses of this group, and there is a real possibility that the vaccinia virus we use today may be a stabilized hybrid between smallpox and cowpox viruses. Whatever its origin, it has some of the same antigenic determinants as smallpox virus and, despite a century of controversy on the matter, no one today doubts that recent successful vaccination provides a very high degree of protection against smallpox and that properly used vaccination of contacts can be depended on to limit and eventually extinguish any outbreak of smallpox.

At the immunological level, Jennerian vaccination is a very simple procedure. Basically it is just a limited attack of smallpox in which the virus multiplies locally and passes to the lymph nodes of the region. A small amount of virus probably always leaks through into the blood when the person has his first vaccination. In the local lymph nodes and elsewhere, antibodies against the antigenic components of the virus are produced and, perhaps more important, clones of cells emerge which can react with some of these. The combination of cellular and humoral (antibody) immunity is sufficient to ensure that when smallpox virus enters the body it will be effectively dealt with by the same sort of reactions that prevent the vaccination lesion from spreading, quite rapidly eliminate the infection, and reduce the pock to a tidy scar.

Such a description begs a lot of questions. We do not really understand why and how experience of one infection allows effective prevention of a second, but the lack of that knowledge is of no practical importance in most circumstances. It is only when we come to inquire into the rare catastrophes that follow vaccination that we begin to see the complexities that lie behind the normal uneventful sequence of a successful vaccination.

In a tiny proportion of vaccinated infants, less than 1 in 100,000, the "pock" that forms a raised whitish bladder on the fifth or sixth day does not dry up to the normal scab but breaks down to an ulcer with an inflamed edge which goes on spreading and enlarging without any sign of healing. The virus is present and active in the ulcer and may cause other infections elsewhere on the body. About 50 percent of these infants can be cured by giving them concentrated human gamma globulin prepared from the serum of people who have been recently vaccinated. Apparently their antibody-producing mechanism is overwhelmed by excess of antigen but they have basically no serious weakness. If the absence of antibody can temporarily be overcome by its artificial administration, the defenses of the body can, as it were, get their second wind and this time function effectively.

But antibody is by no means the whole story. Too large a proportion of these cases of spreading vaccinia do not respond to antibody and end in death. There seems to be another weakness in addition to failure of the antibody response. Then we have the children with no antibody and no possibility of making any — the agammaglobulinemics. Most such children can be vaccinated — or have been vaccinated before their abnormality was recognized — with a normal course and no complications. But among the bad cases that sometimes appear, a few are in children with agammaglobulinemia. These can be minor or major genetic abnormalities of every aspect of bodily function and in all probability the very, very rare severe or fatal illnesses that can follow vaccination nearly all indicate the existence of some genetic anomaly. Probably the most important is the inability to develop the cellular reactions which give the so-called delayed hypersensitivity. Anyone who has been repeatedly vaccinated has seen a manifestation of delayed hypersensitivity in the swift course of an "immune reaction." A primary vaccination takes 2 to 3 days to appear and 8 to 10 days to pass its acme. In the immune reaction there is a sharp red spot by next morning and at 2 days the red papule is nearly as big as it ever will be. The whole course is virtually complete in a week. This accelerated course and rapid healing is currently interpreted as a cellular reaction to antigens of the virus, of the same type as any other delayed-hypersensitivity reaction.

In Britain, America, and Australia, diphtheria is a virtually extinct disease — most of us believe because of immunization with toxoid. There is only one aspect of modern practice in diphtheria immunization that calls for further comment. This is the almost universal use of a preparation of toxoid adsorbed on a precipitate of aluminum hydroxide or some similar insoluble carrier. This improves the production of antitoxin, both in experimental animals and in human beings. The use of "adjuvants" is widespread in experimental immunology, and much more efficient ones than aluminum hydroxide are available. The commonest procedure is to emulsify the antigen solution in liquid paraffin and add killed tubercle bacilli, but this is too irritant for use with human vaccines. The action of the adjuvant is complex, but probably its most important effect is to lay down a depot of antigen from which the actual antigen is only slowly liberated. At the same time there is an active accumulation of macrophages and lymphocytes to the area with formation of plasma cells and much actual production of antitoxin from this local cellular accumulation. On any theory by which cells are stimulated to activity by contact with antigen, there are great advantages to be gained by slowing down and prolonging the presentation of antigen to the cells.

The production and successful use of the Salk vaccine can be held to mark the final, and perhaps the greatest, achievement of preventive medicine against infectious disease. A good deal has been said about the Salk vaccine on previous pages and in this chapter we need discuss only the current attempts to replace the formalin-killed Salk vaccine with a live-virus vaccine to be given by mouth. To be acceptable as a "live vaccine," the chosen strain of virus must combine ability to multiply in the body with absolute inability to produce paralysis. There are several such strains of polio virus covering each of the immunological types, which have been undergoing large-scale tests in the last four years (1958–1961). There is no doubt that these vaccines can produce effective immunity and many millions of children have been vaccinated without any record of paralysis that could be ascribed to the vaccine virus. Some virologists are still unhappy, however, about the possibility that one or other of the vaccine strains may produce paralysis in a very occasional *adult* who had escaped all natural infection with polio viruses during childhood.

The standard course of three injections of Salk vaccine is effective in preventing polio because the antibody provoked will block the virus as it passes through the blood on its way from intestine to spinal cord. The alternative method of immunization insofar as it aims at preventing paralysis has essentially the same rationale. In using live attenuated virus as a vaccine, the objective is that it should multiply in the bowel, producing enough antigen to result in an effective stimulus for antibody production. If the antibody level in the blood can be raised and maintained at an adequate level, we should expect just as satisfactory protection against paralytic disease as with Salk vaccination.

Other factors, however, come into the picture. Some, such as the finding that while one intestinal virus is active in the bowel it may "interfere" with the action of a vaccine strain, are not immunological in character and need only be mentioned. From the immunological angle the most interesting feature is the existence of intestinal immunity which is not seen after Salk vaccination. This is demonstrable by feeding attenuated virus and determining over how long a period it can be isolated from the feces. In a nonimmune individual or a person immunized by Salk's method, virus will usually be excreted for 2 to 6 weeks. In a person naturally immune, or immunized previously with attenuated virus of the same type, virus does not become implanted and is found in the feces for only a few days.

The interpretation of this bowel immunity is still controversial, but there has been at least one demonstration that polio antibody may be present in the bowel and it is reasonable to believe that following intestinal infection there is an accumulation of competent lymphocytes and plasma cells in the various lymphoid accumulations in the region. There are innumerable lymphocytes and plasma cells in the intestinal wall, some loosely scattered, others in centers of lymphocyte production in the appendix or distributed over much of the small intestine as what are called Peyer's patches. Many of the lymphocytes seem to pass into the bowel cavity and it seems highly probable that antibody produced in the same areas also passes into the intestine. The internal surface of the intestine is an elaborate structure of close-packed leaflike projections, in some ways resembling the pile of a velvet. Lying over the tips of these projections is a thin sheet of mucus which serves to lubricate the passage of the contents and prevent damage to the living cells. Any antibody exuding into the intestine would accumulate beneath the mucus sheet in such a position as to bathe the free surface of the intestinal cells. Here it is clearly in a highly favorable position to prevent infection of the wall by any viruses that had found their way into the contents of the intestine.

Immunity in relation to surgical transplantation

In several chapters we have referred to skin grafting as something which is successful only between individuals of the same genetic constitution. We have also mentioned the special occasions when, as a result of an experiment of nature or of a scientist's manipulations, this limitation can be overcome.

Surgeons are necessarily interested in the possibility of transplanting a healthy organ to replace one destroyed by disease. The need is most frequently seen in relation to the kidney. There are several conditions which in young or relatively young people may lead to progressive disease in both kidneys, with failing function and inevitable death. At least four such patients are now alive because they were identical twins with a living partner who was willing to donate one of his own healthy kidneys and undergo the severe operation which that gift entailed. It is technically possible now to take out a kidney and to link it up by artery, vein, and ureter to the appropriate vessels and urinary bladder in a new recipient. In an hour or two it can be secreting urine in normal fashion. If it comes from an identical twin it can continue to function normally, but on the few occasions that other types of donor have been used the kidney has always failed in roughly the same way that a rejected skin graft breaks down.

Plastic surgery can do wonders by making use of the

patient's own tissues to repair damage and loss, but its powers would be greatly extended if tissue from a relative or volunteer, or for the matter of that from the body of a healthy person killed by accident, could be used. In this section we shall discuss some of the surgical possibilities and some of the experimental work on which such thoughts are based. It is an interesting story but it is perhaps wise to say at once that there is no immediate likelihood of success. Even the most optimistic and courageously experimental of surgeons will find that Nature fiercely defends the integrity of the body for all the excellent reasons we have already discussed.

There is only one foreign tissue that can be transplanted with a good probability that it will continue to function indefinitely. This is the transparent tissue of the cornea on the front of the eye. The cornea is beautifully transparent because it contains no blood vessels. This is probably also the reason why it can be transplanted.

As far as we know, corneal cells differ from one person to another in the same way that skin cells do. They are not rejected because the cornea is the one place in the body where the conditions needed for rejection do not obtain. In the first place, the foreign antigenic patterns in the absence of blood and lymph vessels will not pass readily to regions where they can be recognized as foreign. More important is the fact that if immunologically active cells and antibodies are provoked the absence of blood vessels does not allow them to reach the foreign tissue. Corneal grafting is a delicate operation requiring meticulous technique, for the simple reason that if the region is damaged or infected inflammation will lead to the development of new blood vessels and once these reach the foreign tissue the normal rejection process is very likely to begin.

In every other situation we are dealing with tissue which

must have a capillary circulation if it is to survive and we must confront the difficulties squarely.

There are no real possibilities of making use of the principle of tolerance induced by embryonic or immediately postnatal injection of cells from a potential donor. I have heard one surgeon wonder aloud whether it would be worth while to inject a few million of the father's leukocytes into every baby on its first day of life, so that a skin donor would be available if the child should suffer a very extensive burn. A few tests have been made to see whether babies with Rh disease who have received exchange transfusions are subsequently able to accept skin grafts from the donors of blood. The results have been negative. If a means of allowing surgical grafting of foreign tissue is to be developed, some other procedure will have to be found.

In 1960 the most hopeful approach seemed to be based on the use of x-rays to destroy the body's power to react against foreign substance.

To understand the possibilities it will be necessary to describe some of the experimental work on transplantation in more detail than we have done previously.

The effect of x-rays on immunity

It has long been known that if one gives an animal a heavy dose of x-rays it will die. The dose of x-rays is measured in units based on the power of the rays to loosen electrons and ionize air or any other form of matter. The basic unit is the roentgen (r) and we can omit necessary qualifications and speak of a whole-body dose of 400 r. This will result in the death, within 30 days, of about 50 percent of mice so irradiated. If we raise the dose to 850 r all mice will die, the deaths occurring from 5 days onward. It appears that death is largely due to infection from the intestine and the absence of normal defensive mechanisms. The irradiated animal can make no antibody and almost all its lymphocytes have been destroyed.

Lethally irradiated mice can be saved if they are given an adequate number of cells from the bone marrow of a normal mouse. If we are dealing, as will always be the case in serious experimental work, with pure lines of mice, it will be found that, though isologous bone marrow (from the same type of mouse) gives the best results, the immediate response to cells from a different strain is almost equally good. Since we are primarily interested in what happens with cells that are not genetically the same as their new host, we can concentrate on the situation that arises when strain A is lethally irradiated and saved by the injection of bone-marrow cells of strain B. By choosing proper strains, one can distinguish between single A and B cells by their chromosome pattern during mitosis.

The first result is the colonization of the depleted lymphoid tissue by B cells. Since all of A's lymphoid cells have been destroyed or damaged by the irradiation, there is no reaction against the foreignness of B cells and they establish themselves and take over all the functions of mesenchymal cells. They are tolerated by the A host, but we must remember that they are B cells to whom some of the chemical patterns of A are alien. If the association is to be permanent, not only must A tolerate B but B must become tolerant of A. Sometimes this happens. A mouse can go along happily, all of it genetically A except for its mesenchymal cells in bone marrow, spleen, and so forth, which are B. The mouse appears healthy and we can test it for tolerance by appropriate skin grafting. It will accept both B and A grafts. The presence of B cells can be shown in several ways. In some combinations it is possible to show that the gamma globulin circulating in the blood has been made by the transplanted B cells. Two other methods are by examining chromosomes or by inoculating spleen or bone marrow into a normal A mouse and testing this 2 weeks later with a B skin graft. The B cells will provoke an immune response and the B skin graft will be rapidly rejected with a typical accelerated response.

Mutual tolerance is not, however, the only or even the commonest result. Particularly with some combinations the more usual result is a graft-versus-host reaction like those that occur in infant mice similarly inoculated. The mice lose weight, develop a low-grade diarrhea, and die with very small spleen and thymus. In these the A mouse is tolerant to B cells and as long as the animal survives it can be grafted with B skin, but the active B cells have not become tolerant to A. Here obviously is a serious potential danger if similar procedures are to be used with human patients.

There is a third possible outcome. The B cells establish themselves and become tolerant to A but gradually the residual A cells recover and begin to multiply. Without any particular crisis the two mutually tolerant types of mesenchymal cell A and B compete for survival and, probably because they have a better over-all adaptation to their home territory, the A cells gradually oust the aliens. Eventually the *status quo* is restored. There is, however, one observation on such mice of particular interest. The A cells which finally reoccupy bone marrow, spleen, and thymus are descendants from a very few surviving cells, all damaged by heavy radiation. In some mice it is found that a high proportion, in one instance up to 95 percent, of dividing cells in any of the three locations all show a single type of chromosomal abnormality. This can only mean that they are all derived from a single surviving cell. Such a conclusion also establishes directly what has been long suspected, that there is a common potentiality in mesenchymal cells by which in appropriate internal environments they can give rise to red blood cells and the whole range of leukocytes as well as the lymphoid cells of the tissues. One of the main future problems of cell behavior in the body is to find what triggers the direction that development takes.

Before leaving the effect of x-rays, we should mention some experiments in which irradiation was used to cure leukemia in mice. The common form of mouse leukemia is an unrestrained proliferation of lymphocytes which otherwise closely resemble the normal cell. They are highly susceptible to destruction by x-rays and in some experiments it was possible to cure mice by lethal irradiation followed by injection of bone marrow from normal mice. The method is not very reliable. It needs a very large dose to kill all of 10^{10} or 10^{12} malignant cells and even in the best experiments cure did not exceed 50 percent. A minor increase in the malignancy of the strain of leukemia used resulted in a subsequent experiment giving no survivals whatever.

There have been much discussion and some preliminary applications in surgery of these experimental findings. It is highly unlikely that they will ever allow the transplantation of a healthy kidney from an unrelated donor, but, as the difficulties are only (only!) technical, they may be eventually overcome. For the present most of the interest is in regard to the treatment of leukemia and of the rare patients who have accidentally received a gross overdose of radiation in the course of work in atomic reactors and the like. No one has yet claimed to have cured leukemia by heavy x-irradiation followed by bone-marrow transfusion, but it is not impossible that by a combination of chemotherapy to provide a preliminary reduction in numbers and heavy irradiation a proportion of successes might be obtained. The real danger that irradiation of the intensity needed would significantly increase the likelihood of various types of malignant disease in later life would be disregarded in treating a condition otherwise bound to be fatal within months.

A related use of bone-marrow transfusion is to increase the admissible intensity of x-ray treatment for widespread malignant disease. In such cases it is possible to let the patient provide his own bone-marrow cells to be stored before the irradiation and reinjected as a prophylactic measure afterwards.

Tissue scaffolding

There is a form of surgical transplantation which has a rather lowlier function than those we have been discussing. Fairly early it was found that for repair of bone or of the wall of a large artery the corresponding tissue from an unrelated donor could be used. It has gradually become clear that in both instances the important function of the graft was to provide continuing mechanical strength during the period needed for the patient's own cells to get rid of the donor's cells and rebuild viable tissue of the patient's own type on the scaffolding provided by the surgeon.

Theoretically there is much to be gained by eliminating such transplants if a mechanically effective scaffolding could be provided from other sources. Most arterial surgery now makes use of artificial walls woven of synthetic fibers without antigenicity which can be infiltrated by the patient's cells to make a strong and permanent arterial wall. It has been a continuing quest by surgeons to find the most satisfactory materials to leave embedded in a patient's tissues. The reaction to foreign bodies, even of inert materials, has many resemblances to an immune reaction and we may well find that the most suitable material is an organic polymer, all of whose surface groupings are of a type well known to the recognition mechanisms of all human beings.

11. Allergic Disease

Hay fever is a disease of civilization and drug sensitivity is the bugbear of modern medicine. Each represents a reaction of immune mechanisms against foreign material, but distorted for one reason or another so as to produce disabilities which may range from a minor nuisance to fatal disease.

The point has already been made that the immune mechanism which has evolved in man must necessarily be a compromise arrangement whose functioning gives the best over-all chance of survival against the common and important types of infection. When new circumstances and substances come into the human environment, they have to be dealt with by the mechanism that has developed through a million generations of mammalian evolution. This is by no means equivalent to saying that they are therefore dealt with in the manner most convenient and comfortable to the individual encountering them.

Hay fever

Hay fever is seen only in human beings. There are experimental imitations that can be produced in animals but most research on this type of allergy has necessarily to be done on patients and volunteers. The general picture of hay fever is familiar to everyone. If he is not himself susceptible he will undoubtedly have a friend or two who show typical symptoms at the right season of the year. Like most Australians who suffer, I am sensitive to the grass pollens; if I had been brought up in America I would probably include ragweed pollen as well. In a typical example of grass-pollen sensitivity, the subject will show his first symptoms about the beginning of summer — early June in England, the end of November in Australia. The symptoms are inflamed and itchy eyes, sneezing, and nasal obstruction, with occasionally a touch of asthma. The intensity of the symptoms clearly depends on the extent of one's exposure to grass pollen. Hay fever vanishes on any cool, wet day.

Grass pollen contains a variety of substances and most diagnostic studies are made with pollen extracts prepared in a weakly alkaline solution. The active principle in ragweed, the most extensively investigated pollen, is a small protein or polypeptide with a molecular weight around 5000. The standard diagnostic procedure is to make a series of light scratches on the skin and then place on each scratch a drop of one of the suspect pollen extracts. Positive reactions appear within a minute or two in the form of an itchy wheal surrounded by a pink "flare" due to dilatation of the small blood vessels. The reaction closely resembles a mosquito bite, for the excellent reason that a mosquito-bite lesion is actually an indication that the individual has been sensitized to a protein in mosquito saliva. The effect can be imitated in most details by injecting a trace of histamine or putting a drop of histamine solution on a fresh scratch. The sting of a nettle contains histamine, which is responsible for most of the features of a nettle rash.

Antibody in the blood of hay-fever patients is not usually detectable by any conventional test-tube method, but it can be demonstrated by passive transfer to another person (see page 44). In addition to showing that the allergic individual has a specific antibody in his blood, this type of test establishes another important point. Unlike classical antibody this particular type of antibody adheres firmly to some or all of the tissue cells with which it is brought into contact. Its presence on the cell surface is recognized by the histamine liberation from such "sensitized" cells which follows contact with antigen. There is little evidence that any other agent than histamine is concerned in the reaction, and the symptoms of hay fever can all be accounted for on the assumption that they result solely from the liberation of histamine at the various points where pollen or soluble antigen derived therefrom can come into contact with cells carrying antibody. Since 1944 a new and popular class of drug has emerged, the antihistaminic, which by one means or another prevents liberated histamine from producing its usual effects. On the whole, a modern histamine-blocking drug will give almost complete relief from hay-fever symptoms, with a rather variable likelihood of producing in addition some unwanted side effects such as drowsiness.

All this is straightforward and accepted by everyone. The most interesting questions, however, are hardly ever asked and have not been answered. Why do some people and not others get hay fever and why has hay fever apparently become so much commoner in the last 50 years?

There is undoubtedly a genetic predisposition to allergic disease, but we have as yet no real indication of the nature of the actual biochemical lesion. It may be that the essential feature by which the allergic antibody (reagin) differs from classical antibody is the ease with which it can be attached to cell surfaces and render the cells susceptible to damage, at least to the extent of liberating histamine, by contact with the appropriate antigenic determinant. One reasonable suggestion is that the specific reactivity is the same in both types of antibody but that the types differ in regard to the rest of the globulin molecule. It would be very interesting, for instance, to know whether reagins contain the easily crystallized globulin fraction present in classical antibody from the rabbit. Since it is known that the same individual can produce both types of antibody and that some persons seem never to produce the reagin type while others produce reagin even in response to diphtheria toxoid, one is forced to develop a picture of two (or more) populations of cells whose relative importance may differ from individual to individual and perhaps at different times in the same individual. We have only sketchy notions on the nature of differentiation and clonal inheritance among somatic cells, and it seems hardly worth discussion whether we are concerned here with differentiable clones or with cells of the same clones producing different types of antibody according to the nature of the internal environment in which they find themselves.

The association of hay-fever symptoms with the mucous membranes of the nose and eyes makes it natural to think of the possibility that antibody produced predominantly by accumulations of lymphoid cells under the moist linings of various parts of the nose and sinuses would have this character. On other pages we have mentioned, or will mention, special qualities of immune responses arising by entry of the antigen through the skin and through the intestinal lining. The facts available in each case are selected and incomplete and no one has yet made an effort to look at the general significance of differences in the route by which an antigen approaches the body. Until the experimental and observational findings have been elaborated and analyzed, it is hopeless to attempt any broader interpretation at the evolutionary level.

Sensitivity to drugs and other simple chemical substances

Even if we cannot fit them neatly into the biological picture, there is much of immunological as well as human interest in the flood of hypersensitive reactions of all sorts that modern industrial chemistry has inflicted on us. Bakers develop dermatitis of the hands when an "improver" is added to yeast; workers with penicillin may suffer from asthma; "home permanents" produce skin rashes or deodorants lumpy skin in the armpit; and patients develop alarming symptoms from drugs which at first benefited them. However, not all the agents producing hypersensitivity are synthetic: poison ivy produces its characteristic effects only in that proportion of people who develop susceptibility after being exposed to the agent.

Nor do all undue susceptibilities to drugs depend on immunological processes. There is an antimalarial drug, primaquine, which in a small proportion of genetically predisposed individuals interferes with certain enzymes in the red cell in a way which leads eventually to the production of severe anemia.

Immunologic or allergic forms of hypersensitivity are extremely numerous, but two characteristics render them difficult to discuss in general terms. First, they are not seen in all subjects apparently exposed to the same amounts of the agent, and second, the manifestations tend to vary widely in different individuals. Reactions to penicillin may range from some local swelling at the site of injection, or a mild blotchy rash, to fatal kidney damage. In some patients sensitive to penicillin, antibodies can be detected in the blood, and some give an acute wheal-and-flare reaction to a skin test with penicillin. Most, however, show neither.

The example we shall take, therefore, is the experimental production in the guinea pig of skin hypersensitivity to a simple chemical, 2,4-dinitrofluorobenzene (DNFB), which is also a potent producer of hypersensitivity in man. If a dilute solution of this in some bland oil is applied to an area of skin on a normal guinea pig, nothing happens. If the procedure is repeated, contact begins to produce a red patch of inflammation and soon an extreme degree of sensitivity is evident. Substances which can produce this type of response all combine readily with protein and everything indicates that some form of combination with a body protein is a necessary preliminary to sensitization. It is of particular interest, however, that, if DNFB or the similarly active compound picryl chloride (P) is combined with rabbit-serum protein, the complex when purified can be used to produce typical antibody in the guinea pig but it does *not* produce skin sensitivity. If we feed the substance P to guinea pigs, no sensitization is produced but the animal becomes nonresponsive. Contact with P does not now produce skin sensitivity, injection of P-protein complexes does not give antibody.

Serum from a sensitized animal will not confer sensitivity on a normal guinea pig but lymph-node cells can do so with ease. Even if a guinea pig is rendered incapable of active response to the chemical on the skin by feeding P, it can be given a temporary hypersensitivity by this transfer of lymph-node cells from a sensitive animal. Clearly, as in delayed hypersensitivity (see Chapter 4), the cells are the important factor. The unimportance of antibody is also shown by the fact that children with agammaglobulinemia can become sensitized with DNFB and their cells can transfer sensitivity to normal children.

These phenomena have not made the impact upon immunological thinking that their importance deserves and they have not been discussed in any detail from the standpoint of immunological theory. Several points of interest arise when we examine the findings from the point of view of the clonal-selection theory. As an example, we may take the various phenomena observed in guinea pigs which have been treated with picryl chloride (P). According to the clonal-selection theory, there are in normal animals a limited number of cells preadapted to react with the antigenic determinant P. They are presumably located in various parts of the body, where they represent a minute proportion of the cells in various accumulations of lymphoid tissue. The substance P as such is not capable of stimulating these cells. It must be combined with one or other body component if it is to be effective and the nature of this complex plays a major part in determining what reactions follow. If the reported results are taken at their face value and logically interpreted, we might say:

(1) When P unites with some unknown substance x after being given by mouth, Px reacts with *all* the cells in the body that can react with P and either renders them nonresponsive or eliminates them.

(2) When P unites with substance S in the skin, PS stimulates preadapted cells in such a fashion that they multiply but cannot be further stimulated to plasma cells or at least not by PS. Sensitivity arises when a sufficient number of lymphoid cells with the right label have been developed by the animal. As such cells reach an area where PS is present they will be damaged by reaction with the antigen and in the process liberate the agents which cause the red patch of inflammation on the skin.

(3) When P unites with substance A, which may be one of the serum proteins, PA behaves like an ordinary antigen. Lymphoid cells are stimulated first to multiply and then to be converted to antibody-producing plasma cells by contact with PA.

This covers all the main phenomena reasonably well, but no doubt other interpretations are possible. In any discussion of hypersensitivity phenomena, we are worried by the difficulty of deciding between a cell which can react with antigen because it has a genetically determined power to do so and a cell which might be just as reactive because it has absorbed onto its surface an antibody molecule that was produced by some other cell. It is well known that a proportion of antibody molecules, especially those of the hay-fever (reagin) type, can be taken up by cell surfaces and confer upon them some types of reactivity with the corresponding antigen. It is not wholly inconceivable that some types of plasma cell produce antibody which has such an avidity for the surface of lymphocytes that it is whisked out of the circulating blood as fast as it enters. There is another related hypothesis that has to be considered, particularly in relation to work by Lawrence on the transfer of sensitivity to tuberculin in man. This is that a clone of cells which for genetic or other reasons produces antibody specific for tuberculin or some similar antigen may be able to transfer to other cells not only susceptibility but the capacity to produce more of the sensitizing principles.

I believe that most immunologists will be rather unhappy if either or both of these types of process have to be invoked to explain the broad facts of sensitization. But the possibility cannot yet be excluded, and without attempting to discuss details it is easy to see how deeply it might be necessary to modify the simple clonal-selection viewpoint if these secondary processes play a major part.

Sedormid purpura

As a final example of allergic disease with some interestingly different aspects, we may take sedormid purpura. Sedormid is the trade name for a sedative drug once rather widely used; purpura is the medical name for a rash made up of many small or large hemorrhages into the skin. There are a considerable number of cases on record where a patient after taking ordinary doses of sedormid developed a purpuric rash, with or without evidence of internal hemorrhages as well. Blood examination showed a great diminution in the number of platelets.

The platelets are the most inconspicuous of the formed elements in blood and are hardly heard of except among hematologists. They are nonnucleated fragments of cells present in large numbers, 2–5×10^5 per cubic millimeter, and having important functions in dealing with the local emergency that arises at the site of every injury to the body. They are necessary components of the process of blood clotting and of the temporary closure of damaged blood vessels. They are immunologically reactive and may be damaged when an antigen-antibody reaction takes place in their presence with subsequent liberation of histamine, 5-hydroxytryptamine, and heparin. Sedormid is harmless to most people, but in some it unites with the platelets and by so doing becomes antigenic. When antibody reaches an adequate level in the blood, the possibility of a three-body interaction develops. Platelet plus sedormid will interact with antibody to destroy or damage the platelet, and when platelet numbers are sufficiently depleted every minor hemorrhage into the skin or tissues will be checked with increasing difficulty. Clumping and disintegration of platelets can also be shown in the test tube, but again only when the three components are present. Provided the patient's serum is used as the antibody, it is immaterial whether the platelets come from him or from somebody else (Table 8).

There are several other drugs which in occasional patients will produce a basically similar damage by interaction either with the platelet or one of the circulating blood cells. It appears that the drug must make at least a loose combination with the platelet, white cell, or red cell of the blood if destruction of the cells and the corresponding symptoms are to be produced. Some consider that this type of union is also necessary if the drug is to act as an antigen, basing their opinion largely on what has been observed in regard to skin

Table 8. Mechanism of sedormid purpura.

Components *	Interaction	Platelet damage and symptoms
P, S	–P–S	–
P, A	Nil	–
P, S, A	P–S–A	+

* P, platelet; S, sedormid; A, antibody. When damage or destruction of the platelets is beyond a certain degree, skin hemorrhages (purpura) appear.

sensitivity to simple chemicals, as described in the preceding section.

There is, however, an interesting difference. Dinitrofluorobenzene (DNFB) will sensitize everyone who has repeated skin contact with it. Sedormid purpura is very rare among people who have been treated with the drug. This rarity is characteristic of all the "blood-and-drug" anomalies of this group. We naturally think of some genetically determined individuality as being responsible, but as to its nature we can only guess. It is important to emphasize, however, that the variation from the normal is not in the platelet, for that can be replaced by anyone else's platelet, but in the capacity to produce the antibody.

This may be relevant to the current discussions as to whether antibody production is a process of "selection" or "instruction." Instructionist theories claim that the antigen impresses a complementary pattern during the later stages of the synthesis of a globulin molecule, the primary synthesis being genetically neutral. If this is so it would be reasonable to expect that, if a given substance was a good antigen, that is, provoked active antibody production, in one individual, then it should be just as effective in any other individual, or for that matter in any other vertebrate capable of making any antibody. On the other hand, if potential antibody patterns are limited to those produced by some extensive but random process during embryonic life, the existence of a "fringe" of chemical patterns which are antigenic in limited and sometimes very small proportions of the individuals exposed is only to be expected. This individuality of antigenic response is not wholly limited to human beings. It is notorious that rabbits differ in their antibody-producing capacity and mice even more. If an immunologist wants a strong antibody against some substance of relatively low antigenicity, he will always inject at least six rabbits and if none of those satisfy him he will inject a dozen more. He will be disappointed if one of the rabbits does not give a serum far better than the majority.

In recent years much interest has been shown in the possibility of preparing artificial substitutes for blood plasma to be used in conditions of shock or hemorrhage. What is needed is a soluble substance of moderately large molecular size with the physical properties of viscosity and colloid osmotic pressure similar to those of plasma or of serum. There are natural and artificial long-chain macromolecules which have such properties and which have been used in medicine. Their potential advantages are: (1) they can be easily sterilized, (2) they present no risk of producing serum jaundice, a hazard with all transfusions of blood or plasma, and (3) they are nonantigenic.

In fact, however, both of those commonly used, dextran and polyvinyl pyrrolidone, although they produce no antibody in the great majority of people, can produce it in a small minority. It is particularly interesting that one man was found to have dextran antibodies *before* he ever received dextran.

The clonal-selection theory can provide a straightforward interpretation of these findings. In whatever way the primary distribution of immunological patterns is made to mesenchymal cells, some patterns are bound to be more common than others, while some will only rarely be produced. Inevitably, some persons will possess too few cells for a clone of activated cells to emerge as a result of stimulation by antigen.

The existence of a simple interpretation on the basis of clonal selection is, however, by no means adequate to eliminate the possibility of an instructionist theory of antibody production. It might be suggested, for instance, that in order for an antigen to be placed in its final position in an antibody-producing cell it must undergo partial digestion or some other type of modification in another cell. Differences between individuals in ability to produce antibody might then be due not to differences in the actual antibody-producing cells but in the cells carrying out the preliminary stages. As anyone knows who has had close experience of any scientific controversy, particularly in biology, it is extremely difficult ever to produce a set of experimental facts which are unequivocally decisive in favor of one or other side. However much A contends that such and such an experiment proves that the answer is "white," B will always be ready to demonstrate that at most the experiment may show that some shades of gray are possible but that there is nothing in them that positively excludes "all black" from being the real answer.

12. Autoimmune Disease

In Western countries disease resulting from infection and malnutrition now produces only an insignificant proportion of deaths. Prevention of such diseases is essentially routine, and the chief interest of preventive medicine has necessarily turned to those diseases which are intrinsic to the individual and not directly due to the impact of the environment. Until a hundred years ago infectious disease, particularly in childhood, and particularly in undernourished children, was the major killer. Today it is our pride that children are well nourished, protected by one means or another against infection, and educated. The death rate is low and the expectation of life at birth steadily increasing — but hospitals seem to be as full as ever.

Our medical problems now are still to a considerable extent environmental in origin. With each important social development new medical problems seem to arise. Automobile accidents have become a major cause of death; prosperity, overfeeding, and a sedentary life have heavily increased death from coronary disease; cigarette smoking has made lung cancer the commonest type of malignant disease in men; and it seems that each new technical advance in industrial chemistry must be paid for in the early stages by a crop of poisonings. Perhaps the most important segment of disease today is mental illness of various types. Much of this is genetic in origin, or at least has an important genetic component. How much functional nervous disease is directly referable to social environmental difficulties, or how the relative genetic and environmental effects should be assessed, proves a great and probably insoluble problem for preventive medicine. None of these have much direct relation to immunity.

The residuum of medical problems includes essentially those conditions which are intrinsic to the individual and which in most cases must be interpreted as genetically based deviations from the average. In many, perhaps most, instances, the deviation will be manifested in disease only if appropriate environmental factors reinforce the genetic weakness. A boy with hemophilia is likely to bleed excessively only if there is an actual injury, a cut or a tooth extraction, for instance, to initiate the hemorrhage. Length of life is to a very considerable degree an inherited quality and the converse of this statement must also be true, that a majority of fatal illnesses in persons over middle age have an important genetic component.

The commonest problem in medicine is to understand how the sequences of processes, genetic, environmental, and what we may call physiological, cooperate to produce an illness which may or may not be diagnosable in terms of conventional pathology but which shortens life.

We have so far said very little about genetic aspects of immunity apart from talking a good deal about somatic genetics in relation to clonal selection and mentioning on several occasions the existence of agammaglobulinemia. In this chapter, however, we are concerned with a number of anomalies of the processes of immunity which in the last analysis must be based on genetic deviations from the normal. Often all that we can say is that they are disease conditions for which some rare mutation or combination of genes must provide the background without any opportunity for closer genetic analysis being possible. What is possible is to study some of the processes which intervene between the genetic anomaly and the full pathological manifestations of the condition. Here we are most likely to find a means both of analyzing some of the processes operative in normal individuals and of finding ways to modify the pathological process therapeutically.

The combination of biochemical and genetic studies on bacteria, fungi, and other microorganisms has provided a powerful tool to determine how the actual processes of biochemical synthesis proceed in the cell. The famous generalization "one gene, one enzyme" is at least near enough to the truth for us to assume that where a detectable change in bodily function can be shown by genetic tests to be due to a single gene mutation, we shall find on adequate study that somewhere a single definable chemical step has been blocked or distorted. It is equally reasonable to expect that when unitary genetic changes arise, either in the germ cells or in the (somatic) cells of the body, which cause immunological anomalies we may expect the nature of these anomalies to throw important light on the steps by which antibody is produced and immunity established.

Congenital agammaglobulinemia has so far been the most revealing of such anomalies. This inherited disease, limited to males and until the antibiotic era always fatal, has been briefly described in Chapter 4. Here we need only state summarily that the key disability seems to be an innate inability to produce plasma cells. Without plasma cells there can be no antibody. On the clonal-selection theory this means that all behavior is normal except that there is no way in which an immunologically competent cell can be stimulated to become a plasma cell. Somewhere there is a functional block which prevents contact of antigen with an appropriately preadapted cell from initiating the normal physiological switch to the plasma-cell form.

In some ways the most interesting, and from the human angle the most distressing, feature of these children with agammaglobulinemia is that when, as a result of careful watching in hospital and the skillful use of antibiotics and normal serum, the child survives for several years, he almost always develops joint troubles of the general quality of rheumatoid arthritis. More rarely he may show symptoms of one or other of the *autoimmune* diseases.

It is still by no means clear why these children should develop autoimmune disease, but the fact that they do provides a convenient starting point for the discussion of this group of diseases. Since in agammaglobulinemia antibody in the blood is never produced, we can feel sure that rheumatoid arthritis and the other so-called autoimmune diseases are not primarily due to anomalous antibody production, even though it may be easy to show in most cases that abnormal antibodies are present. But before we become too much concerned with the primary character of *cell* changes in autoimmune disease we should probably try to define the meaning of the term autoimmune.

Irrespective of how antibody-producing cells arise in the first place, most immunologists would be willing to agree that in the adult human being (or other mammal) there are many clones of cells carrying the potentiality of producing one or other antibody, plus a smaller number of clones actually producing some antibody. There are, however, in the healthy person no clones producing antibody directed against components of the body. One way of defining autoimmune disease is to say that a disease condition is autoimmune when it can be shown that signs and symptoms are being produced by the direct or indirect action of clones of immunologically competent cells (including antibody-producing cells) on antigenic determinants carried by normal body components. Up to the last year or two the only way of establishing the existence of such clones was to demonstrate autoantibodies in the blood. There are signs that a more fundamental approach, in which primary attention is paid to the cells, will eventually be possible.

As in other chapters, no attempt will be made here to discuss autoimmune disease in medical or technical detail. The objective will again be to use the phenomena to help elucidate the nature of the immune process. The diseases to be considered are rheumatoid arthritis, rheumatic fever, acquired hemolytic anemia, and a chronic disease of the thyroid gland named after a Japanese physician, Hashimoto's disease.

Of these, rheumatic fever and rheumatoid arthritis are the only ones likely to be known to the layman but the thyroid condition is the easiest to understand.

Hashimoto's disease of the thyroid gland

Hashimoto's disease is a chronic swelling of the thyroid gland with at first rather indefinite symptoms that eventually take on the classic picture of lack of thyroid hormone — thickened, puffy skin and slowness of thought and movement. If a piece of the thyroid is removed and examined microscopically the most conspicuous feature is an invasion by lymphocytes and plasma cells, neither of which are present in a normal thyroid. Within the last 3 years it has been found that in these cases the blood contains antibody against one or both of two thyroid-gland components. One of these is thyroglobulin, a protein specific for the thyroid gland, which is stored in the saclike follicles of the gland. The other is less well defined but forms part of the finely granular material (the microsomal fraction) of the actual thyroid cells.

The current interpretation of the disease is that it results from the development of an immune response against a part of the body which lies, as it were, outside the stream of everyday traffic among the expendable cells of the body. There are some organs which are not commonly subject to damage and in which worn-out cells are not dealt with by phagocytosis. Their essential components seem to be broken down as necessary and released into the blood in a non-antigenic form. Though there may be a number of components sufficiently different from those common to all body cells for them to be potential antigens, these remain *inaccessible* under normal conditions.

The actual initiating cause of Hashimoto's disease is unknown. Some suspect that a more or less accidental bacterial or viral infection may cause local damage in the thyroid; then, if the person concerned is abnormally weak in the faculty that we can call immunological control or homeostasis, a vicious-circle process can be initiated. At the site of damage thyroid antigens can pass out and lymphocytes and other mesenchymal cells can move in. Whatever the process by which immunologically competent cells arise, after a certain extent of antigen leakage from the thyroid such cells are present. Some take the form of plasma cells and release antibody into the blood. Others are attracted to and invade the thyroid, finding there the specific stimulants which will both result in the production of tissue-damaging agents and cause proliferation of some of the stimulated cells. This increase in local damage increases release of antigen and entry of cells, and unless some other factor intervenes the logical result is continuation of the inflammatory damage until the thyroid is a burnt-out relic without hormonal function.

The condition can be imitated in the rabbit by surgically removing half the animal's thyroid, grinding this up with a suitable adjuvant mixture, and injecting it into the rabbit that provided it. In a few weeks the rabbit shows both the cellular invasion in the thyroid and antibodies in the blood. There is, however, one highly significant difference. In the experimental animal the process is self-limited and, despite the initial invasion of the thyroid by inflammatory cells, the function of the gland is not seriously impaired and within some months the organ becomes histologically normal. The continuing process in the human patient clearly needs some additional, presumably genetic, weakness in immunological control.

There are several important lessons to be learned from Hashimoto's disease. The first is the concept of the "inaccessible" antigen which is so segregated from the rest of the body that there is no need for it to be "on the list" of self patterns against which antibody production is forbidden. Second, we can recognize clearly the capacity of cells with appropriate immunological competence to inflict tissue damage on organs containing the antigenic patterns that correspond. Then we have the vicious-circle character of most such reactions; damage is necessary to initiate immunological response, which itself inflicts more damage, which allows more immunological response, and so on. Finally, if the current interpretation is correct, that the damage to the thyroid is due essentially to the action of immunologically competent cells rather than to any effect of antibody in the blood, then we must always be careful to regard antibody more as an indication of the existence of active cells than as a cause of organ damage and symptoms.

Of rather different character is the fact that after all Hashimoto's disease is a rare one, recognized, as a rule, only by specialists in thyroid disease. Yet it is obvious that many people can have a transient damage to the thyroid without developing Hashimoto's disease. If our picture of a vicious circle was the whole story, everybody's thyroid would be in a highly vulnerable condition. As soon as any damage was received an irreversible process of chronic inflammation and destruction would be initiated. Since this is not the case, we must postulate that in the immunological field, as in every other aspect of bodily function, there are built-in controls, homeostatic mechanisms analogous to those that see to it that when there is too much CO_2 in the blood a whole series of physiological responses come into play to bring it back to normal level.

In Chapter 7 we mentioned one possible way by which any clones of cells that were directed against body patterns could be eliminated. This was based on the assumption that when a cell was stimulated by an antigen to proliferate it passed necessarily into other physiological states, in some of which further contact with antigen was highly damaging. When an antigen is always present in the environment, there cannot be antibody production or proliferation of any sort of immunologically competent cells.

There are probably other more subtle mechanisms at present unknown. One which has been studied, particularly in relation to the resistance of mice to the transfer of experimental cancers, is of some general interest. This is that the presence of antibody against a certain antigen, whether of intrinsic or extrinsic origin, may render immunologically competent cells of the same specificity inert. Suppose a damaged thyroid is leaking small amounts of antigen T into the tissues and the blood. If there are appropriately reactive lymphocytes in the body, any reaching the thyroid area in blood capillaries or lymph paths will make contact with the antigen and produce their damaging effect. If, however, antibody against T is circulating freely in the blood there is every probability that there will be no effective amount of free T in the thyroid region to attract active cells there. This may be one of the reasons why quite a large proportion of hospital patients with other types of thyroid disease, and some without any evidence of thyroid trouble, show antibody of the same general character as is found in Hashimoto's disease. It reminds us, too, of the fact that children with no antibody and without any potentiality of producing antibody are highly prone to a mild form of rheumatoid arthritis.

Rheumatoid arthritis

Let us therefore take rheumatoid arthritis as our next example of autoimmune disease. It is only gradually that this interpretation has come into vogue and it is still uncertain how the autoimmune process is related to the joint changes. There are two main pieces of evidence. In the first place, rheumatoid arthritis responds, temporarily at least, to treatment with cortisone, prednisolone, and other of the corticosteroid drugs. Without quite knowing why, most physicians now consider that if a condition responds to treatment with these drugs it has an important autoimmune component. Conversely, if it does not respond we should look for some other type of diagnosis. The second line of evidence is more direct. The serum from a rheumatoid-arthritis patient very often shows an unusual globulin which can be demonstrated by a variety of what might almost be called laboratory tricks. The commonest is to treat sheep red cells with antibody just short of the amount that will cause them to agglutinate. In this semistable condition they will be rapidly agglutinated by the globulin found in most rheumatoid sera but not in normal serum.

A more sophisticated approach shows that the rheumatoid factor is an unusually complex globulin molecule and that it reacts with damaged (denatured) human gamma globulin. This is a particularly interesting situation immunologically because antibody is itself gamma globulin and when an antibody reacts with its corresponding antigen it will usually be progressively denatured. So we have the possibility that an antibody against some determinant pattern in denatured gamma globulin will, by reacting with the antigen, itself become the same antigen. Here obviously is another possibility of a vicious circle being brought into being. Equally obviously, most people must possess an inbuilt protection against the possibility of developing the vicious circle.

In the inflamed joints of rheumatoid arthritis, there are abnormal accumulations of soft tissue (synovial villi) which under the microscope contain numerous lymphocytes and plasma cells. A recent application of fluorescent-staining techniques to this problem has allowed some of these cells to be functionally identified. A suitably prepared solution of denatured globulin can be chemically labeled with a fluorescent dye. It then becomes a specific stain for any cell containing antibody against denatured gamma globulin, which is the same as saying that it stains cells producing or containing the rheumatoid factor. Many of the plasma cells in sections of diseased joint tissues when so stained give a bright fluorescent glow under the microscope and in some of the lymph nodes there are centers of lymphocyte production which show the same evidence of being produced for a special function. Perhaps it is equally important that not all the plasma cells in the diseased joint tissues fluoresce and that most of the centers of production in lymph nodes are uninvolved.

Most pathologists would say that it is still too early to interpret these findings, but in a book like this one there is nothing to be gained by refusing to risk being wrong. No textbook would ever be written if the author insisted that nothing he says could ever be made out of date by future research. What we have to say about the nature of rheumatoid arthritis will certainly be proved incomplete and possibly turn out to be wholly wrong. But to say it clearly is the best way of accelerating the effort to gain a *better* understanding.

We believe then that rheumatoid arthritis is a disease due to the reaction of immunologically competent cells with certain body antigenic patterns that are present in the tissues of the affected joints. One of the most important of these patterns is carried by denatured gamma globulin, but this is probably a secondary rather than a primary phase. It remains for future research to find what are the other patterns that attract damaging cells to the joints and the accessory conditions that are necessary to bring the unwanted immunological activity into being. One might guess that there is a genetic element. For one thing, rheumatoid arthritis, like most autoimmune disease, is more frequent in women than in men, and there is some direct evidence that arthritis runs in families. For many years it was thought that chronic infection in the tonsils or elsewhere played a part. This view of "focal sepsis" is now mostly dismissed as an ancient medical superstition, but, in view of the considerable resemblances between rheumatoid arthritis and rheumatic fever, we should perhaps keep something of the sort in mind. Somewhere we may need an area of lymphoid tissue under the stress of chronic infection to allow the first emergence of those forbidden clones of cells that are going to plague the patient. This concept is something that can be better discussed in regard to rheumatic fever.

Joints, particularly the small joints in the hand, are subject to knocks and strains, to heat and cold, and one pictures the process starting at some point of casual damage. The patient is predisposed genetically to weak control of her immune reactions, and one assumes that a few "forbidden" cells are already in existence ready to react with components made accessible by the initial damage in the joints. Once started, the process can build up progressively, but we must remember that it is a process which can go on only because of some little-understood weakness of control. Once that control is regained, the process must stop, though past damage may not necessarily be repairable.

Cortisone is known to the public mainly as a cure for rheumatoid arthritis, and this is perhaps the best place to say something about the corticosteroid drugs and the salicylates. Both can provide great symptomatic relief but they have no effect on the basic mechanism of the autoimmune diseases and in that sense are not curative. In neither case do we know precisely what the drug does. It seems, however, that, though the corticosteroids like cortisone and prednisolone are weight for weight immensely more potent than the salicylates (including aspirin) and have many additional effects, their essential action in autoimmune disease is the same. Nothing we know is inconsistent with the view that corticosteroids (and aspirin) act by *diminishing the response of an immunologically competent cell when it meets the corresponding antigenic pattern*. Cortisone and hydrocortisone are natural hormones which almost certainly play a part in maintaining and adjusting the size and distribution of the main population of immunologically competent cells in the body — the lymphocytes. When we know more we shall almost certainly find that they have a major role to play in the control processes that prevent the emergence of forbidden cell clones or render them harmless when they do appear. It is not unreasonable therefore to find they are therapeutically helpful. To be slightly more specific — but it is still only a guess — the structure of the corticosteroids suggests strongly that they should act on the cell surface and we can picture their action as modifying the surface of the lymphocyte so that it fails to respond to what should serve as a trigger to action. With an increase in the dose of corticosteroid, lymphocytes are selectively destroyed. The diminution in response therefore may be merely the first stage in a process of general damage to the lymphocyte.

Perhaps it should be pointed out here that the capacity of a natural hormone to destroy selectively one type of normal cell is unique and points to a special function of the lymphocyte that makes it necessary for its numbers to be changed abruptly as circumstances require. In Chapter 7 we related this to the hypothesis that lymphocytes were the main carriers of immunological information. Most physiologists prefer to think more materially of the lymphocyte as a mobile and easily accessible source of the components of protein and nucleic acid that may be needed for any emergency. The two concepts are in fact complementary. If there is need to produce rapidly a new population of cells of one immunological character, it is obviously convenient to call on unwanted cells of similar type to provide the building stones from which the new ones can be built. All lymphocytes are made of the same bricks and mortar; they differ only in details of pattern. Any lymphocyte could be cannibalized to help build any other type of cell that was needed.

Rheumatic fever

Rheumatic fever is a result of streptococcal infection of the throat and tonsils. If we prevent streptococcal infections we will see no rheumatic fever, nor will we see any typical cases of acute nephritis in children. In one sense, therefore, we are dealing with something which is just as much an infectious disease as measles or polio. In medicine, however, we can never be content with the simple statement that a disease x is caused by y. Usually we will discover that though y is a necessary factor it is not in itself a sufficient cause of the disease. In addition we have always to face the problem of pathogenesis, the process by which cause or causes interact with bodily processes to produce the symptoms of which the patient complains and the changes that the pathologist finds in the organs.

In rheumatic fever we always find a preceding streptococcal infection, but that infection has nearly always become quiescent before the child or adolescent suffers his attack of rheumatic fever. The typical disease comes on rapidly and causes severe pain and exquisite tenderness in the joints, with high fever. It has no resemblance to a streptococcal infection of a joint, and everyone is agreed that the streptococcus as such plays no part in producing the symptoms. The delay of 1 to 2 weeks from the height of the streptococcal episode to the onset of joint symptoms points rather strongly to an immunological process, and there are at least two possible interpretations of what happens. The most popular is that in the throat the streptococci produce a soluble product which if we like we can call a toxin. This toxin enters the blood and passing round the body is taken up by cells in the joints and occasionally in other parts of the body. The toxin is antigenic and after a week antibody begins to appear in the blood. The antigen, however, is still present in the joint cells, and when the antibody reaches a sufficient level it reacts with the antigen there and produces the characteristic symptoms. It would perhaps be more in line with modern ideas to speak of the emergence of immunologically competent cells capable of reacting with the streptococcal toxin and to ascribe the lesions to an invasion of the joint tissues by such cells instead of ascribing the whole reaction to antibody.

The alternative is a more subtle one. It assumes that the reaction is autoimmune in character. We have already given the evidence that part at least of the rheumatoid reaction is due to reaction with altered gamma globulin, and there is much to suggest that rheumatic fever is essentially a more acute form, in a younger individual, of the process that produces rheumatoid arthritis in the middle-aged and elderly. If this is so, the function of the streptococcus must be indirect. Perhaps the fact that only streptococcal infections *of the tonsillar region* produce rheumatic fever indicates that a modification of lymphoid tissue by streptococcal infection can in some way allow the production of cells directed against bodily components. In Chapter 7 we assumed that there was always the possibility of a mesenchymal cell clone arising which could react against a body component. Since the great majority of body components will be in every cell of every tissue, any such cell arising in spleen or lymph node will be subject to stimulation and control of the type we discussed. The present suggestion is that, for reasons still to be elucidated, immunologically competent cells of one or a few types can proliferate in a tonsil infected with streptococci although they would be eliminated at once in a normal person. If large numbers of cells reactive against component x are liberated into the blood, and if component x is most readily accessible in the joint linings, we have a means by which symptoms can be initiated. If, in addition, we bring in the requirement that reaction between antigen and competent cell produces local damage which makes more antigen accessible and available to react, then we have an immediate explanation of how a chain reaction can build up and produce the full-blown picture of acute rheumatic fever. We do not know that this explanation is the true one and we have no indication as to the nature of the tissue antigens involved. Most people will probably prefer the streptococcal toxin theory until a definite decision becomes possible by the isolation of the antigen. It should be emphasized that both the streptococcal toxin of the first hypothesis and the tissue antigen of the second are products of imagination and logic. They have not been experimentally identified and may not exist.

There is one condition observed, particularly in the wards of infectious-disease hospitals, that mimics rheumatic fever fairly closely and throws some light on its nature. This is serum sickness. A child is given a big dose of diphtheria antitoxin, which is essentially purified horse-serum globulin, and when its diphtheria has vanished nicely it rather suddenly develops fever, a blotchy rash, and painful sensitive joints. This condition appears at the same time as laboratory tests show that antibody against horse globulin is appearing in the blood. The explanation is the same as that offered by the streptococcal-toxin theory for rheumatic fever. The foreign globulin lodges in various tissues, including skin, joints, and kidney, and, as the blood antibody rises, reaction with tissue antigen produces the various symptoms. The difference from rheumatic fever is that despite the large amounts of antigen involved in serum sickness the local symptoms are much milder than those of rheumatic fever.

Before leaving rheumatic fever, we should mention that there have been attempts to combine the best points of the two hypotheses by assuming that the streptococcal product combines with a cell antigen to produce something which can stimulate cells to make antibody which will react both with the combination and with the same antigen in its uncombined state. This is, however, a cumbersome compromise that can have no virtues until the more logical theories are *both* proved to be inadmissible.

Acquired hemolytic anemia

This is a disease or a group of diseases which are characterized by an acute destruction of the red blood cells with resulting anemia. Sometimes it follows an obvious bacterial or viral infection; more often it is recognized after a period of vague ill-health.

Acquired hemolytic anemia was the first of the autoimmune diseases to be recognized as such, and since the red cells are primarily involved it is one of the simplest to study in the laboratory. There are many variations in the immunological findings but it will be enough to describe those of the most straightforward group. There is first the evidence from anemia, excretion of blood and bile pigments, and enlargement of the spleen that red cells are being actively destroyed. The blood is found to contain antibody of rather weak character (incomplete antibody) which agglutinates the patient's red cells and those of most normal individuals. A detailed study of which red cells are and which are not agglutinated by the patient's serum will sometimes show that the antibody reacts with one of the Rh series of antigens, most often e, but the majority of sera appear to react with a pattern common to all human red cells and therefore never found in blood grouping investigations.

Appropriate tests will show that the circulating red cells are partially coated with antibody. This antibody is, of course, globulin and its presence can be detected by testing the cells with a serum against human gamma globulin made by immunizing a rabbit. A positive result is shown by agglutination of the cells — a positive Coombs test. The hemolytic anemia is ascribed essentially to this coating of antibody which results in the premature destruction of the red cells in the spleen. The antibody obviously is something which should not be there, a forbidden antibody in every sense of the word and derived from a forbidden clone of cells.

Acquired hemolytic anemia is of crucial importance for the understanding of immunological processes, if only because the phenomena are almost completely inexplicable on the classical instructionist theories. Here there is no question of an inaccessible antigen; thousands of millions of red blood cells with all their antigens are made and destroyed every day. The antibody produced is not stimulated by or directed against some peculiar antigen on the patient's own cells. It is equally active against most other human red cells, both in the test tube and when the test is made with cells labeled with radioactive chromium in the body. It is particularly significant that the antibody is usually one which is never produced when cells from one person are transfused into another. It is concerned therefore with a pattern that is universal to all human beings — or, to be more accurate, to all but one or two families with the rare blood-group anomaly designated technically as (–D–/–D–). It is clearly one of the first antibodies whose production is forbidden by the process of progressive self-recognition that goes on during embryonic life.

On the clonal-selection theory the essential lesion in acquired hemolytic anemia is the appearance of a forbidden clone of mesenchymal cells and its failure to be suppressed by the normal control (homeostatic) mechanism. When we look closely at this hypothesis, several new problems arise. If a forbidden clone can arise against body antigen A, then it should also be possible for clones against B, C, D, and so on also to arise. By hypothesis, the readily available antigens will stimulate the corresponding forbidden clones to proliferate instead of inhibiting or destroying them. Why then do we find in this disease only one type of abnormal antibody in most cases? Probably no fully satisfactory answer can be given, but it seems probable that it will eventually be found to be related in some way to the function of the spleen. In hemolytic anemia the spleen is enlarged, and in some cases, at least, removal of the spleen will cure the disease. Histological section of the spleens removed at operation show, as would be expected, active phagocytosis of red cells by the macrophages of the spleen. This is reasonably ascribed to the antibody coating on the surface of the red cells, but we should perhaps remember that there is one case of acquired hemolytic anemia on record in a boy with congenital agammaglobulinemia. He was cured by removal of the spleen, which showed much red-cell phagocytosis. This is almost the only piece of evidence that macrophages can manifest specific reactivity against a particular antigenic pattern.

To fit the facts our hypothesis could be elaborated to assume (1) that the multiplication of, and antibody production by, the forbidden clone can take place only in the spleen or (2) that stimulation of the clone requires the pattern in a partially broken-down form which can be produced only in the spleen. This means that the breakdown in homeostasis is not a general one but is confined to some function of the spleen. There is a rather strong suggestion that what happens in the spleen in acquired hemolytic anemia may be very similar to what happens in the tonsil in rheumatic fever.

Systemic lupus erythematosus (SLE)

Only physicians are likely to have heard of what is a rather rare disease usually involving women and sooner or later fatal. Systemic lupus erythematosus is usually referred to in the clinics as SLE or just lupus. It got its name with the recognition that a certain type of rash on the face was liable to be associated with symptoms involving many regions of the body, notably the joints and the kidneys.

The only reason for mentioning SLE is that it is the auto-immune disease par excellence in that the forbidden immunological activity is directed against the most vital of all cell components, the DNA of the nucleus. Very little is really known about how SLE is produced; undoubtedly there are genetic factors concerned, and one gets the impression that most of the subjects are predisposed and the disease is only waiting to be triggered by some relatively minor infection. In its full-blown form the symptoms and the changes that can be shown by laboratory tests in the blood both point strongly to the conclusion that a wide variety of forbidden clones are active, many of them liberating antibody into the blood.

The blood serum in SLE is extremely interesting to an immunologist. There is an abnormally large amount of gamma globulin and there are a great variety of reactions against body components. Some physicians are chary of ascribing these reactions to antibodies, but this seems to be mere prejudice. Physically, the reactive globulins are antibodies. They appear to be antibodies that correspond to a variety of configurations associated with the cell nucleus. The first to be described was an antibody which could cause a degeneration of cell nuclei that could be easily recognized under the microscope. Cells which have engulfed such damaged nuclei are known as LE cells and are an important diagnostic sign of this and some closely related conditions. There are several other sorts of antibody, but we need refer only to that which reacts with DNA. As every biologist knows, deoxyribonucleic acid, DNA, is the key substance for all life above the smaller viruses. It is the substance that carries the genetic information of the cell and is the material basis of the chromosomes. It is probably correct to say that there are no chemical differences that could be recognized immunologically between DNA's from organisms as different as bacteria and men. The only "different" DNA is found in a group of bacterial viruses, and it is highly significant that the only antibody to DNA that has been produced in a normal animal is against this unusual form.

In the body, cells and nuclei are always being broken down and DNA must be free in various stages of disintegration within, for example, the germinal centers of lymph nodes. If for some reason the normal body veto against cells or antibody that could react immunologically against normal body components is relaxed and cells capable of reacting with these nuclear fragments including DNA are present, there is clearly plenty of "antigen" available to stimulate proliferation of such cells and antibody production. The most likely interpretation of SLE is that, for some reason basically genetic, forbidden clones of cells appear which can react with a wide variety of body components. This must open the way for what may quite legitimately be referred to as a chronic civil war within the body. The damage produced by the forbidden cells and antibodies may be temporarily diminished by the careful use of corticosteroid drugs and there is some evidence that the spontaneous partial recoveries which occur may also be due to these same hormonal substances produced by the body itself.

Medically, SLE is a disease of extreme interest and in the last decade many hundreds of papers have been written about it. For our purpose, however, its importance is as a condition in which forbidden cells and antibodies can flourish and be directed against a configuration common to every cell of every animal. It is not therefore an inherent quality of cells to be incapable of reaction against their own constituents. Here is probably the strongest argument in favor of the clonal-selection approach. Antibody can be produced against DNA and virtually every other of the body's components, but in every normal man or animal there is a regulatory (homeostatic) mechanism to ensure the elimination of all such patterns as they appear.

One may conclude this brief and superficial discussion of the autoimmune diseases by emphasizing the way in which they all point to a modification of immunologically competent *cells* by which they become insusceptible to normal controls. Only a theory couched, like the clonal-selection theory, in terms of the population dynamics of body cells can at present provide the necessary framework for generalization. If the phenomena of autoimmune disease are to be considered from an "instructionist" point of view, that theory will need to interpret (1) the nonantigenicity of body components, (2) the possibility of a breakdown in that nonantigenicity, and (3) the nature of the homeostatic mechanism preventing such breakdown in the normal individual.

13. The Deeper Problems

Immunology is not yet fully integrated into the pattern of general biology and perhaps it is foolish even to think of such an integration until we have gained more subtle understanding of several important biological fields than we have at present. Nevertheless it seems not inappropriate to end a book of this type with some highly personal speculations about how immunology may in the future both help the gradual formation of the elusive integrated picture of biology and be interpretable in terms of wider concepts.

In the first chapter we took as a starting point the necessity that every multicellular organism must protect itself from infection by pathogenic microorganisms and that the form taken by immunity following infection in the higher vertebrates, including man, had clear survival value. This is probably self-evident, but when one tries to bring protection against infectious disease into relation with the various phenomena that are related to self-recognition, and with which this book has been mostly concerned, one meets serious difficulties. There is no special reason why the evolution of defense against infection should necessarily involve an elaborate self-recognition mechanism.

Very little really is known about immunity in invertebrates, except that antibody formation does not occur and that, at least in larval forms, there is a relatively wide acceptance of grafts from generally similar organisms of distinct species. The elaborate mechanism with which we have been concerned seems therefore to be a relatively late development in evolution, especially associated with vertebrates. For these and a variety of other reasons, biologists have sought another approach to the evolution of immunity, starting with the idea that self-recognition in the broad sense is primary and anti-infectious immunity something that was superadded later on. This is an approach that necessarily takes us into rather deep waters, but maybe it is worth the plunge.

It is a truism that the raw material of evolution is mutation. There is usually a very complex process before any mutation that brings something new of survival value to the species is in a position to make an effective contribution. Deleterious mutations and other inheritable errors and anomalies in the germ cells may, however, be rapidly eliminated. The only feature that need be emphasized is that there is a potentiality of error in every replication of the genetic machinery of every cell. Undoubtedly some genetic systems are more prone to error than others, but there is sufficient evidence to make it likely that at any given genetic locus an error in replication occurs with a frequency in the range 10^{-5}–10^{-7} per replication. This must introduce an important additional requirement into the processes needed to maintain cellular integrity in a large multicellular organism such as man, with probably more than 10^{14} cells constantly reproducing, including such short-lived cells as the lymphocytes. There must be many millions of errors (mutations) occurring every day of our lives, and complex and long-lived multicellular animals could not have evolved unless some means of dealing with this eventuality had been developed.

As I have discussed at length elsewhere, the most rational explanation of malignant disease is that it develops when somatic mutation or some equivalent process produces clones of cells whose potential for differential survival exceeds what can be tolerated by the body as a whole. Where mutation in any given direction is likely to occur with a frequency of only about 10^{-6}, the efficiency of the tissue in which it occurs will not be significantly modified unless it is a mutation which by reducing the responsiveness of the cell to normal controls allows it to proliferate more effectively than its congeners. The most satisfactory interpretation of the age incidence of cancer is that malignant change emerges as a result of a sequence of mutations within a cell line, each of which adds a certain proliferative advantage.

Mutations outside this field will in general be undemonstrable clinically, but as they accumulate with age we should expect a gradual failure of efficiency in bodily function. Any somatic-mutation theory of aging will need a great deal of elaboration and experiment before it can be accepted; on the other hand, what other type of theory of aging is available? Perhaps the most persuasive argument in its favor is that irradiation of mice at relatively low levels shows a significant shortening of average life span without seriously modifying the pattern of pathological changes found at death. All this is only relevant to our present topic insofar as it justifies the assumption that somatic mutation in large long-lived animals is a factor of importance in relation to survival.

It is part of current dogma that any mutation that has a detectable result will involve at some point the production of a protein of different structure from the normal. This depends on the well-accepted teaching that a change in the genetic information carried by DNA in the chromosomes is transferred via RNA to protein (usually an enzyme) as the first step toward the appearance of any phenotypic effect. Replacement of one or more amino acid residues in a protein will potentially, at least, allow it to be recognized by immunological methods as different from the original form. This leads us to our hypothesis that within the body there has developed a means for the recognition of potentially dangerous somatic mutation, and that this is the basis on which the immunological functions of the vertebrates have been evolved.

To support such an evolutionary hypothesis we should, if possible, provide: (1) an indication that somatic mutation is or can be harmful to survival; (2) evidence that the mechanism suggested can serve to prevent or reduce this harmful effect; (3) an indication where new experimental evidence should be sought to support or disprove the hypothesis.

We have already shown that somatic mutation, particularly to malignant disease, does provide a threat to survival and we can therefore concentrate on the second and third requirements.

There is no doubt that in man there is a wide variation in the invasiveness, and conversely in the curability by standard procedures, of malignant disease. On rare occasions histologically verified cancers have retrogressed, with prolonged clinical cure. Much more frequently standard surgical and radiological treatment of cancer provides more than 5 years' survival that could not be expected if every cancer cell had to be removed or killed to achieve this. The body seems to have some resistance of its own against some developed cancers. It has been reported that when the histology of gastric cancers removed at operation is studied a positive correlation is found between the intensity of the lymphocytic response and postoperative survival. It is only a hint, but it does point to the possibility that a "homograft-immunity" type of response can on occasion be provoked by a spontaneous tumor. The evidence from experimental tumors is not specially relevant to this point, but it is axiomatic that a spontaneous tumor will in almost every case be transferrable only to isogenic individuals. In all others the transplanted tumor will retrogress under the impact of an immunological response.

The only other types of somatic mutation that are clinically recognizable are those occurring at relatively early stages in embryonic life. From the previous discussions of prenatal tolerance, it will be evident that these could not be expected to provoke any type of immunological counter. Nonproliferative types of somatic mutation in adult life may be common and may be dealt with immunologically, but the possibility has never been and perhaps never can be explored. It is, however, legitimate to claim that there is evidence that immunological reaction could do much to counter the type of harmful effects that somatic mutation may produce.

A hypothesis that does not suggest and call for experiment is scientifically useless. If somatic mutation is constantly occurring, one would expect to find, particularly in older individuals, small amounts of antibody against the most frequent of the mutant patterns. The only way of guessing what the most frequent mutants might be is to assume that somatic mutation will produce the same sort of changes as are known or presumed to have arisen by germinal mutation. The only area open to experiment is in regard to blood groups. One might expect that, in a person genetically defined in relation to perhaps eight different sorts of blood groups, somatic mutation among the stem cells from which his red blood cells are derived might produce a tiny proportion of cells of mutant type and that some of these mutants would be to a type known to occur in other individuals. Such an occurrence might be recognized either by the appearance of unexpected "spontaneous" isoagglutinins in the serum or, more likely, by a selective response to one particular antigen when a small injection of a foreign blood is given. Some exploratory experiments along these lines in Australia have so far given negative results. This is only to be expected, but if the possibility is kept in mind it may sooner or later provide an explanation for an otherwise inexplicable antibody or clinical reaction.

Our hypothesis then seems to be reasonably acceptable on the three primary criteria, and with an improved knowledge of the types and nature of somatic mutation opportunities for further experimental test should increase. There are, however, some further requirements which are at least desirable in regard to any hypothesis couched in evolutionary terms. It is not very helpful to postulate a quality — in this case capacity to recognize chemical differences between self and not self — however valuable it might be for survival, unless the quality in question can be derived in some reasonable fashion from some more general and primitive quality.

Very recently there have been a number of indications that immunological recognition may be derived from an aspect of the processes by which all multicellular animals succeed in maintaining a characteristic morphological and functional unity. In its most general formulation this capacity must involve an interchange of "information" between cells. A cell seems to be able to "recognize" whether another cell is in contact with it or not and in some instances whether the adjacent cell is of its own type or another. For the appropriate reactions to take place, which allow, for instance, the reconstruction of a traumatized area into something functionally and morphologically equivalent to its previous normal form, one must postulate a rather elaborate structure of effector and receptor patterns, chains of stimulation and of feed-back controls. Effector and receptor patterns as factors in morphogenesis have been sponsored by Weiss for many years, with a mutual relation of antigen-antibody type. Here then is a potential basis on which a specialized recognition function of lymphoid cells may have been evolved.

One of the objections to this point of view was the generally accepted opinion that the immunologically important cells were short-lived, wandering cells, accumulated admittedly in various regions of the body but not themselves concerned with any morphological function and showing no indication of ever having been related to morphogenetic cells in the course of their embryonic development. It is too technical a matter to elaborate, but it is significant that at the present time the possibility is being canvassed that the lymphoid cells concerned with immunological functions are derivatives of intestinal-type epithelium rather than of primitive mesenchymal cells. The earliest cells of thymus, tonsil, and a specialized "tonsil" at the wrong end of the intestinal canal in birds (bursa of Fabricius) are epithelial, and some histologists are now claiming that the lymphocytes which subsequently appear are descendants of these epithelial cells.

All this is rather thin speculation and it may appear foolish to attempt to interpret immunology in terms of embryonic differentiation and morphogenesis about which we know very little. Information and ideas must, however, flow back and forth between the different areas of biological research, and a hypothesis linking immunological recognition on the one hand with embryonic differentiation and morphogenesis on the other may be helpful to both.

The hypothesis that immunological recognition has been evolved from and has remained part of the control system by which the body maintains its structural and functional integrity is no more than a hypothesis. But it is in accord with the whole trend of modern immunology that it should be true. At the present time the requirement is for much more information in regard to cellular aspects of immunity, with a rather special need to extend immunological studies beyond the common experimental mammals of the laboratory. It is not always an advantage that biological research should be almost wholly supported by money earmarked for medical or agricultural research. If one could hopefully dream of an affluent society in which war, infectious disease, malnutrition, and overpopulation had been overcome, biological research could still provide an infinite field for the exercise of effort, ingenuity, and intelligence. And when we are freed from the obsession that biology is concerned only with disease, there may be a special urge to use the ideas now arising in immunology to help unravel the processes that maintain the integrity of the body. In the end we may find that only by this route we come back again to the problems of disease from which both the name immunity and the science took their origin. Infectious disease as a practical problem is conquered, but it will remain endlessly interesting to go on searching out the how and why of that conquest.

Bibliography

The following is a very limited list of recent works on immunology from which detailed access to the literature can be gained. A few important papers on immunological theory are also noted.

General texts on immunology in English

Chapters in René J. Dubos, *Bacterial and Mycotic Diseases of Man* (Lippincott, Philadelphia, ed. 3, 1958).

W. C. Boyd, *Fundamentals of Immunology* (Interscience, New York, ed. 3, 1956).

Topley and Wilson's *Principles of Bacteriology and Immunity* (Edward Arnold, London, ed. 4 by G. S. Wilson and A. A. Miles, 1955).

Special topics

R. R. Race and R. Sanger, *Blood Groups in Man* (Blackwell, Oxford, ed. 3, 1958).

M. F. A. Woodruff, *The Transplantation of Tissues and Organs* (Thomas, Springfield, Ill., 1960).

H. S. Lawrence, ed., *Cellular and Humoral Aspects of the Hypersensitive State* (Hoeber, New York, 1959).

F. M. Burnet, *The Clonal Selection Theory of Acquired Immunity* (Vanderbilt University Press, Nashville, Tenn.; Cambridge University Press, Cambridge, England, 1959).

Papers on theories of immunity

L. Pauling, "A theory of the structure and process of formation of antibodies," *J. Am. Chem. Soc. 62* (1940), 2643.

N. K. Jerne, "The natural selection theory of antibody formation," *Proc. Nat. Acad. Sci. 41* (1955), 849.

D. W. Talmage, "Immunological specificity," *Science 129* (1959), 1643.

J. Lederberg, "Genes and antibodies," *Science 129* (1959), 1669.

F. M. Burnet, "The mechanism of immunity," *Scientific American 204* (1961), no. 1, p. 58.

Index